Caring for My Mom

with Love, Laughter, and Tears

A Journey Through Caregiving
at the End of Life

Rae Ann McKeating

Caring for My Mom with Love, Laughter, and Tears
Copyright © 2013 Rae Ann McKeating

Published by End of Life Issues
ISBN: 978-0-9891449-0-2
LCCN: 2013935105
Cover design and chapter image by Jacque Burton

Printed in the United States of America

The author of this book does not dispense medical advice or prescribe the use of any technique as a form of treatment for physical, spiritual, emotional, mental, or medical problems. If medical advice or other professional assistance is required, the services of a qualified and competent professional should be sought. The intent of the author is to share her experience. In the event you use any of the information in this book for yourself, the author assumes no responsibility for your actions and is not responsible or liable, directly or indirectly, for any form of damages whatsoever resulting from the use (or misuse) of information contained in or implied by this publication.

Because of the dynamic nature of the Internet, any web addresses or links contained in this book may have changed since publication and may no longer be valid. The views expressed in this work are solely those of the author. The names of certain people have been changed to respect their privacy.

This book is in honor of my beloved Mom, Anne

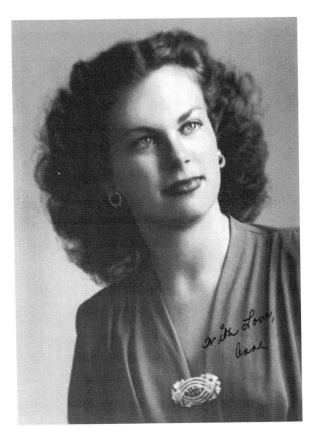

and is dedicated to all those individuals
who work in the hospice field.

Prologue

My Mother was my best friend, my mentor, and my role model. I knew that no matter what I had done or what I had to face, I could always count on Mom. She rarely leaned on me, and, with one exception, she never asked me for help. Her one request took me by surprise when she said, "*I want to die at home with you taking care of me.*"

I could not believe my ears. My mind started racing, screaming out these thoughts: I wasn't a nurse, how could I take care of her? Where would she sleep? How would I handle the emotional strain? She wanted to die in my home. What about my job? What about my life?!

But instead of saying what I was thinking, I gave her a big hug and replied, "Yes Mom, I promise to take care of you at home until...well...I'll take care of you." I must have said those words with a confidence I didn't have, because I saw peace wash over her face before she smiled, held me close, and whispered, "*Thanks.*"

So began our period of learning about death and dying, as together Mom and I waited for her life-limiting cancer to change her body and our lives.

Our lessons came in unexpected ways, sometimes incredibly fast and other times painfully slow. Our journey was not easy, but then journeys through rugged terrain seldom are. Yet given a choice, I would not hesitate to travel that path again,

1

and relive every moment of sorrow, hope, love, laughter, and tears.

With help and guidance from hospice, during those final months I learned how to better care for Mom, allowing her to live each day to the fullest, to say her good-byes to loved ones, and to leave this life as she wished, cared for by her daughter and surrounded by the comforts of home.

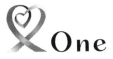

One

Cancer - Round One
September - November 1995

Twenty years after having gone through menopause, my mom began experiencing symptoms similar to having her period. She was a bit concerned, but since the problem wasn't constant, she rationalized that it was just part of getting older. When she eventually shared her symptoms with girlfriends, each one urged her to see her doctor. Mom finally listened, and after a few tests, a uterine cancer diagnosis was confirmed.

I was scared to death, not ready to think about losing a parent, frightened of the unknown path ahead, with no knowledge of how to battle cancer. The next Sunday I bought two small gold angel pins at the Unity Church bookstore, on the slopes of Diamond Head in Honolulu. I immediately pinned an angel on my blouse to remind me that I would not make this journey alone. I believe in a higher power that watches over us and that our life journey is energized through a combination of destiny, luck, and choice. I needed that pin to remind me of my faith.

In early October, Mom, Dad, and I met with a surgeon, whose professional presence and sensitive speech relayed a perfect combination of confidence and compassion. He explained what would happen

3

during her three-hour surgery. Up to that day, Dad and Mom were the parents, and I the child. Although I suggested Mom and Dad schedule the surgery at a time that worked for them, I couldn't believe it when they told me they wanted to schedule the surgery in a few months — just to enjoy planned travel. By then, I had started researching cancer and because I believed cancer is a race against time, I didn't want those damn cells living one extra day in Mom's body. So I lobbied for an earlier date for surgery; they agreed, and we scheduled it for later that month.

Early on Tuesday, October 31 — a Halloween I won't ever forget — Mom had surgery at the USC Norris Comprehensive Cancer Center in Los Angeles. The only other time that Mom had been a patient in a hospital was when she gave birth to me. She was a pioneer of her generation, giving birth to me without anesthetic. That was a clue that she not only had a high tolerance for pain, but that she was mentally strong, a winning combination for the fight ahead.

During the surgery, Dad and I sat together in the hospital waiting room, each pretending to read a newspaper or a magazine. At one point, Dad walked to the cafeteria for another cup of black coffee. I stayed, fearful to miss any updates we might receive. Suddenly, I smelled my Grandma, Mom's mother, and my head snapped around, certain she wasn't there, but needing confirmation that I was correct. I soon realized that the lady on my left, who had just sat down, smelled like Grandma (I bet I could smell Coty Airspun Loose Face Powder twenty rows back in a crowded auditorium). It was a smell that I associated with Grandma's love and memories of seeing that colorful round cardboard box container of face powder carefully placed in the top right hand corner on her bathroom counter. I smiled as I remembered seeing the familiar container during my visit with her the previous week. I took comfort in knowing that Grandma was well cared for at the assisted living home, just blocks from Mom and Dad's house, which made it easy for Mom to visit her several times a week. At ninety-three, Grandma was physically healthy, but due to her dementia we decided not to worry her with her daughter's cancer diagnosis.

Dad returned, handing me a coffee. He said, "I met a retired teacher in the cafeteria checkout. His wife had cancer surgery last week. They've both been pleased with the daily care she's received, and she gets to go home today." After finishing our coffee, we turned back to reading.

Sometime later, I nudged Dad with my elbow. After having looked down the hall for the thousandth time, I finally saw Mom's surgeon walking our way. Still in his green scrubs, he took us aside, lowered his glasses and turned to Dad. "The surgery took longer than expected, but the cancer was contained in her uterus and I got it all out. We'll be moving your wife to the recovery room soon, so wait here, and someone will come to get you when she wakes up."

We thanked him, walked back to our chairs, and sank into them with relief, our bodies relaxing for the first time that day. Silently, we each said a long thank-you prayer.

Mom was in the hospital for seven days. Throughout their forty-nine years of married life, my parents shared one bed; they loved to cuddle. Those seven nights apart were their longest period of separation. Although I am sure neither one liked the time apart, they never complained; complaining was just not in their nature.

We celebrated Mom's seventy-second birthday in her semi-private room, with a cupcake and candle. It wasn't dinner out with friends, but in many ways it was better, with the three of us celebrating her continued life. We were grateful the cancer had been contained and removed, and we were ecstatic that she would soon be up and about, healthy, and able to enjoy life. Our gift was being able to spend more time with her. We sang happy birthday before she made her wish and blew out the candle, then Dad sliced her chocolate cupcake in thirds. With a smile, he leaned over Mom, first to give her a kiss and then to feed her that celebratory birthday cake. We savored each bite, knowing that this was a birthday to remember.

The day Mom was released from the hospital, I gave her the angel pin I had worn, and I started wearing the second angel pin on my outfits. I wore that pin every day for many years. Before her cancer returned, while I was Mom's caregiver, and for years thereafter, the daily ritual of pinning on my angel reminded me of the love I had for her and of the love she held for me.

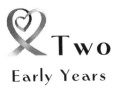

Two

Early Years

My Dad was my hero and I loved him dearly. At eighteen he enlisted in the US Army, serving as a tank commander in the Third Army under General Patton. During four years in World War II, my Dad fought in many battles, had five tanks shot from under him, and lost numerous friends. He lived through hell and suffered through recurring nightmares for more than fifty years.

But nothing prepared Dad for the day he learned Mom's cancer had returned. The thought of living without her was unbearable; she was the glue in our family. Not only was she beautiful on the outside, she was kind, loving, caring, and reliable, a friend to many, and the center of our universe.

Mom and Dad met in the early 1940s, at a dance in Huntington Beach, California. During her "Last Months," as I like to refer to that special period when Mom and I grew even closer, Mom reminisced about meeting Dad:

"I was a student at Huntington Beach High School. I never dreamed I would grow old, let alone get cancer. I loved to jitterbug and swing at the Pavilion on Huntington Beach Pier, which was walking distance from home. My girlfriend Annabelle and I convinced the manager to hire us as coat check girls, saving us the cost of admission; if we weren't busy, one of us would sneak out to dance. One

night I caught the eye of a tall, slender, good-looking boy with dark wavy hair.

I smiled his way, and my heart fluttered when he winked back. He was dancing the Big Apple with a redhead, who turned out to be his sister, your Aunt Doris. She had agreed to drive your father to the dance but only if he would dance with her. Your dad and I laughed about that for years. When we met, I was seventeen and your father sixteen."

On a sunny afternoon the first day of June in 1946, shortly after Dad returned from World War II, my parents were married in the brick Methodist Church in Montebello, California, Dad's home town. Mom often reminisced about how happy she was walking down the aisle, smiling when she recognized a familiar face among the hundred and fifty guests, her four-foot long, lace veil framing her hair from behind. Her satin, floor-length wedding gown cost Grandma and Grandpa most of their life savings, but they didn't care; their only child was marrying the man of her dreams.

Following a short honeymoon in San Francisco, my parents settled in Santa Barbara so Dad could continue his education that had been interrupted by the war. He enrolled at Santa Barbara College of the University of California, starting back to school that summer.

After World War II there was a housing shortage. Like so many other couples at the time, Mom and

Dad considered themselves lucky to find not a house, but one room to rent. They didn't mind sharing the one bathroom with several other couples, nor did Mom mind the inconvenience of having only one shelf in the refrigerator on which to store their groceries as she learned how to cook. My parents were young, deeply in love, and together, ready to take on any and all challenges.

I am a baby boomer — an only child, born in April 1952, almost six years after they married. By the time I was born, Mom and Dad were living in Downey, a city east of Los Angeles and home to one of the earliest McDonald's hamburger restaurants. After graduating from college, Dad began his career in education as a woodshop teacher at Bellflower Junior High School. They had the good fortune to buy a new one-story 1,100 square feet home, which showcased a brick fireplace in a modest size living room, with a kitchen and eating nook, and three small bedrooms on a large 8,000 square foot lot, located in a subdivision with young families just like ours. The fathers in the neighborhood worked while the mothers stayed home and took care of the children. Mom formed friendships with other moms on our block, some which lasted her lifetime. On weekends it was always the three of us visiting family, friends, or playing at home.

My Dad loved change. In a restaurant he would always order the special; on vacations he toured new places. He even convinced Mom to move every five years. I was four when we moved ten miles from Downey to Montebello; I was nine when we moved twenty blocks to a home with a bigger yard. At thirteen we moved twelve miles west to Whittier. Teenagers don't want to change schools, but the move worked out well, and I still am friends with classmates from Whittier High School. In 1970, one month after I graduated from high school, we moved south thirty-six miles to a growing community in Newport Beach. A few years after I moved out, my parents moved twenty miles north to Long Beach. Moving provided the change Dad enjoyed.

Mom and Dad made an attractive couple. At five feet, seven inches, Mom fit nicely under Dad's protective arm. She was pretty, with big blue eyes and a cute, upturned nose. She wore her hair short, her natural curl allowing her to shampoo, blow dry, brush and go, without needing curlers, a curling iron or product. She began coloring her hair when I was ten, perhaps her gift after joining the work force or a necessity to cover annoying gray hairs. Like mine, through the years her brunette hair had been tinted, streaked, weaved, and dyed. I inherited Dad's hazel eyes, good teeth, and his love of change. I have my Mom's smile and her love for Frank Sinatra's music. She idolized him, and to this day I can't hear Sinatra without thinking of her.

By high school, Dad had worked his way into adult education administration and Mom was happy being a bank teller for Security Pacific Bank. Each Saturday morning Dad would go golfing, and before his car backed out of the driveway, Mom had Sinatra playing on the stereo. She and I cleaned house and talked while Frank crooned to us.

My parents enjoyed life, and they continued, through the years, to enjoy each other. They were wealthy, not in dollars, but in their love and respect for one another. Their marriage worked, in large part, because they were good communicators. They talked through problems of all sizes. I'm grateful they didn't know the size of the problem the future would bring.

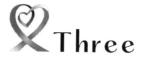

Three

Mom and Dad's Retirement Years

Sometimes talking helped us move through sad times, like when Dad's mom suffered a debilitating stroke. Up to that life-changing moment, fate had taught Nana to be fiercely independent. In 1923, three months after Dad's birth-- when his sister Doris was two--Nana's young husband died suddenly. Overnight she was thrust into the role of provider. She found employment as a high school teacher at Garfield High School in Los Angeles, a position she held throughout her career. During the Depression in the 1930s, she was the sole breadwinner for her two children, her sister, her parents, and her grandparents. At eighty-seven, that cruel stroke left her paralyzed and unable to communicate. She endured a physical prison for more than three years. Her tragic end of life was a reminder to my parents to enjoy each and every day.

The year after Nana's stroke, Dad's colleague died of a heart attack, two weeks after having retired at age sixty-five. His unexpected death caused my parents to discuss the pros and cons of early retirement. They ended up agreeing that because life is short they were willing to sacrifice income and a larger retirement fund in exchange for living each day together to the fullest. They would cut back on spending and concentrate on enjoying life.

So in 1984, when Dad was fifty-nine and Mom sixty, they retired, sold their home in Long Beach, and moved to the Palm Springs area.

It turned out that early retirement was a good choice for my parents. They enjoyed cruises and made new friends at their new home in Monterey Country Club, a twenty-seven hole golf course community in Palm Desert. Dad would golf three or four times a week, while Mom would walk, visit with the ladies, and read by the pool. Both enjoyed sunshine 350 days of the year.

During the years that my parents were relishing their retirement, I graduated from law school and practiced law in California and then Hawaii, where I lived and worked on the island of Oahu. Mom and Dad appreciated having time to visit me on that beautiful island paradise. Together they enjoyed eleven healthy, happy years of retirement before Mom's cancer diagnosis.

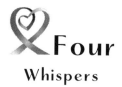

Four

Whispers

After her October 1995 surgery, Mom healed, and our daily activities resumed, except now Mom met with her oncologist every three months. Follow-up care included a physical exam and blood work. The oncologist would check for recurrence (the return of the cancer in the primary site) and metastasis (the spread of the cancer to another part of her body).

Six months after Mom's surgery, I started to hear what I refer to as "whispers," an inner voice suggesting I take a specific course of action. I think of those whispers as my internal GPS; it urged me to move from Hawaii to the mainland to be closer to my parents. I tried to ignore the whispers because I loved living in Hawaii, and I embraced each sunny day with its warm temperatures averaging seventy-five to eighty degrees. I also loved the gentle trade winds that caressed my skin, and I cherished long walks past palm trees lining the bustling streets of Waikiki and the majestic banyan trees, their roots growing in reverse, reaching to the ground from above and providing large areas of cover in the parks. It was a joy to stroll barefoot along the beach, Diamond Head rising in the background, sand between my toes, and surfers on my right. The ocean's vibrant shades of aqua and deep blue that framed the shore never failed to be picture worthy, and occasionally, during a passing rain shower, I would be treated to a dazzling rainbow. The smells from the fragrant plumeria flowers made me smile, as did the respect shown to nightly sunsets. The closer the sun came to setting on the horizon, the quieter we observers would become, until all conversation ceased. Everyone would focus on that day's stunning sunset, which, the moment it slipped out of view, was generally followed by applause.

I am a morning person, so it was a delight to wake at five and enjoy my cup of coffee on the lanai as I welcomed the morning sunrise. At first sunlight, I would join others out for a morning jog through Kapiolani Park and up and over Diamond Head. I appreciated every day I lived in Hawaii.

But if you've heard your own whispers, you know they don't go away; they just get louder and louder. Mine were saying, "Find a job in California; move closer to your parents." So I started looking for work opportunities in California, and by luck, I found an excellent prospect.

In June 1997, I accepted a position as general counsel for a public company with its headquarters in Sausalito, California. By changing jobs, I had traded a five-hour flight from Honolulu to Los Angeles for a one-hour flight from San Francisco to Palm Springs, finally silencing those persistent whispers.

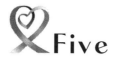

Five

Cancer - Round Two
October - December, 1997

M oving closer to my parents made it easier for us to visit each other. I often flew to see them, but they also enjoyed the ten-hour drive from Palm Springs north through San Francisco, over the Golden Gate Bridge, to my two-bedroom, two-story condo in Mill Valley. It was during their October visit that I asked Mom about her recent oncologist appointment and the results of her tests.

"I guess the results are fine, although the nurse mentioned a big word I didn't understand, something that started with an 'm'. I'm sure it isn't important, but I am scheduled to meet with the doctor the week after we get back home."

A wave of nausea washed over me. I was scared that the nurse had told Mom her cancer had metastasized. Because Mom wasn't familiar with the term and didn't know it meant her cancer had returned in some other location, she hadn't understood the nurse. But instead of screaming "No!" I nodded in agreement and changed the subject, refusing at that moment to acknowledge life's inevitable mortality.

The following morning I cooked bacon and scrambled eggs while Mom set the table and buttered the rye toast. Dad was looking forward to driving into the city for lunch after they had cleaned up the kitchen. We hugged good-bye, and I made the three-mile drive to my office. Once there I closed my office door and called Mom's doctor. Fortunately, Mom had granted permission for both Dad and me to have access to her medical information. I spoke with the nurse, who confirmed my worst fear: Mom's uterine cancer had returned. Tests had revealed that the cancer was now active in her lungs. I vividly recall sobbing as I sat at my desk, visible to all through the glass walls. Stacks of documents piled on my desk-- papers that had my full attention yesterday--were now far removed from my thoughts. How could this be happening to my mom, to our family? I could not imagine my life without Mom, nor could I imagine Dad living without her. It was hard for me to breathe. After giving me time to be alone and regain my composure, my office friends offered hugs and support. (During the months that were to follow, I leaned on them a lot.) I decided not to tell my parents that day, but instead to keep the devastating news to myself; tomorrow would come soon enough.

Later, after arriving home, I changed out of my business suit into jeans, a sweater, and thick socks, happy to free my feet from my high heels. Dad lit the Duraflame log in the fireplace, and as the roaring fire warmed us, we sat in the living room, talking about our day, each sipping a cocktail before dinner. Mom loved her vodka martini with three olives, Dad his scotch and water with a lemon twist. And I, supporting the Napa and Sonoma vineyards, enjoyed a glass of chardonnay.

Mom and Dad had taken advantage of that cloudless, sunny day by making the short four-mile drive to Larkspur, parking their car at the Larkspur Ferry Terminal and riding the ferry to the San Francisco Ferry Building at the foot of Market Street. It was fun hearing my parents' childlike excitement as they described sitting outside on the second deck, the sea breeze playing with their hair, in awe of being so close to the Golden Gate Bridge, the Bay Bridge, and Alcatraz Island. They couldn't stop talking about the stunning San Francisco skyline. After the thirty-minute ferry boat ride, while walking along the Embarcadero to eat on Pier 39, they reminisced about their honeymoon. During lunch they devoured cracked crab dipped in butter and mayonnaise, accompanied by warm sourdough bread smeared with butter, and a few glasses of sauvignon blanc.

Earlier in the week I had made a delicious meat lasagna, so that evening Mom didn't have to prepare the main course. As I was growing up, Dad had insisted that every dinner include protein, vegetable, starch, and salad, even though many nights Mom and I would have preferred a large bowl of buttered popcorn. She did *not* love cooking, a trait I inherited from her. Mom preferred to eat out, but their budget didn't allow that too often.

Most mornings, Dad would ask Mom what we were going to have for dinner, and she might answer, *"We're having baked pork chops, corn, potatoes and a lime Jell-O salad with pears."*

Poor Mom. Ensuring each meal fit neatly into the recommended food pyramid was a bit of a struggle, particularly when her mother-in-law was a home economics teacher. When the menu was announced, Dad would argue, "We can't have corn and potatoes, because those are two starches."

I would have been inclined to reply, "Who cares? That's what we're having for dinner."

But Mom knew how to handle Dad. She was a willow tree, bending to satisfy his every need, except when she absolutely wanted her way—and then of course she was the victor. She would smile: "*Honey, would you prefer potatoes and broccoli?*" Dad would respond, "Yes, that sounds fine." For Mom, the good news was that unless they were entertaining, we rarely ate dessert, so she didn't have to bake many cakes, pies, or cookies.

That evening, while the lasagna was baking, Mom prepared a green salad and served it with garlic bread. Knowing what I knew that night, the drinking part of the evening was easy, but it was hard for me to eat. Talking to Mom's nurse had definitely ruined my appetite.

The next day was Saturday, and Mom and I had planned to go shopping at the mall for clothes and then to Costco for staples. Dad would stay at home to organize my garage and trim and nourish the plants on my patio. Wearing jeans and a sweater, I was dressed for the day. Before leaving Mom upstairs to finish applying her make-up, I told her I would meet her in the kitchen in about ten minutes. I prayed for strength and slowly walked down the stairs to find Dad. It was time to tell him the news. He was in the living room, on his way to the outside patio.

"Dad, do you have a minute?"

"Sure," he replied, smiling as he turned his head to look my way, his right hand opening the sliding glass door.

"Dad, I've got some really bad news. Yesterday I called Mom's doctor to learn the results of her last tests, and it's not good. It's..it's..horrible," I stuttered, holding back tears as I faced him. His eyes bore into mine, urging me to continue. With my voice failing me, I whispered, "The nurse told me Mom's cancer is back. It's in her lungs."

He yelled at me. "You had no right to call her doctor!"

I stepped back, floored by his response. I had expected tears, perhaps a hug, but not a reprimand. In hindsight, I realize that I was just the lightning rod for his anguish, but at the time I was stunned.

"*Is something wrong?*" Mom called down from upstairs.

"No," I quickly shouted back. "Dad and I are fine."

Shaking all over, I quietly asked, "Are you going to tell Mom?"

"Absolutely not," he uttered angrily. "You had to interfere, you tell her." He stepped outside, and slammed the patio door, hard enough to make his point that I was the villain, but not hard enough to upset Mom upstairs.

20

I ran into the kitchen to get as far away from him as I could without running upstairs or going outside. As I slumped into a chair, I couldn't help but turn my head toward Dad. Even from a distance, I could see his back and shrugging shoulders, his head lowered into his hands, sitting on my lone white plastic patio chair, sobbing. Seeing him suffer, and knowing I couldn't make it right, hurt even more than his yelling at me, something he had done but a few times in my entire life.

Dear God, my world has turned upside down, I thought. Dad was supposed to be the one in charge, telling me that everything was going to be okay, and making it all right. Instead, my Rock of Gibraltar had crumbled, and I couldn't turn back the clock. There was no way for me to comfort him, so the next item on my list was to break the news to Mom.

Lost in thought, I didn't hear her come down the stairs. Startled to see her and afraid that she would want to kiss Dad good-bye, I suggested that we say a quick good-bye to Dad and be on our way, as I didn't know how bad the traffic would be. She seemed a bit surprised, but she agreed. We both yelled "Bye," and although he didn't turn our way, we saw Dad's right hand give a feeble wave in our direction.

Maybe Dad's reaction had put me over the edge, but I told Mom the news while I was driving on the freeway, on our way to Costco. Instead of finding a quiet setting and gently raising the matter, I chose to tell her our life had changed again while we were on the road. Clearly, I wasn't thinking at all.

Tears were starting to form as I blurted out, "Mom, I called your doctor yesterday. It's horrible news; your cancer has returned." Answering her unasked question, I added, "I already told Dad."

"*Okay*," she said softly, turning to face me. Then, she reached into her purse, found her coral Revlon lipstick, and began applying it while checking her appearance in the mirror above the passenger seat. I wasn't sure she had heard me.

"Mom, do you understand? Your doctor wants you to see him to talk about treatment—like chemotherapy."

"*Yes honey, of course I understand. I always knew that there was a chance my cancer would return. Sweetheart, remember through the years I have said, 'Right up to this very moment my life has been perfect?' Well, it's still good. I don't feel sick. Your father is healthy, you're healthy, the sun is shining, we have homes, good friends, and we are visiting with you. There's nothing I can do about it today, so don't let it ruin our time together. What is meant to be will be. Honey, life is full of change. Nothing stays the same. Right up to this very moment my life has been perfect, okay? Most of us face health challenges. I'll talk to your father later on. Let's just not think about it now.*"

And so our lives changed; but for a few months they actually stayed the same. Mom decided that she didn't want to start treatment until after the holidays, even though she clearly understood the risk that came with her decision. She and Dad enjoyed a planned cruise with friends, while I immersed myself in work, putting in twelve-hour days, working in the office on Saturdays and from home on Sundays.

The year ended with a Christmas visit from Mom and Dad. Year's end is a busy time for many public companies, so there was no time off before Christmas, but after work I managed to find time to buy and decorate a tree. Although it didn't look as nice as the ones my parents used to dress, its smell said it was Christmas and the extra strands of white lights made up for the deficiencies.

Christmas morning came, and we exchanged presents and laughed when we discovered that each had given the other slippers and a new robe. A family once more, we cherished every moment that day, but deep inside, each of us was wondering if this would be the last Christmas the three of us would ever share together.

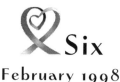

Six

February 1998

Mom started chemotherapy in February, and I flew from San Francisco to Palm Springs to accompany her to the first appointment (as much for me as for her). I had no idea what the term "chemo" really meant, much less how, where, or by whom it was administered.

I remember walking Mom into the large, brightly painted waiting room filled with others who were also fighting cancer. More than twenty chairs were filled with patients of all ages, each at different stages of treatment. Some wore wigs, some hats, and others scarves; some wore nothing on their heads and proudly showed their baldness. I saw patients who looked extremely weak, while others looked very strong. Interestingly, a positive attitude among the staff and the patients was the common thread.

Mom and I were surprised because the "giving" of the chemo was easy—it was the "receiving" that was hard. Mom sat in a comfy, beige suede recliner, with controls that she could adjust to ensure she was in a comfortable position. During her three-hour treatment, as first the IV bag of anti-nausea medicine and then the chemo dripped into the vein in her right arm, she could read, talk, listen to music, watch TV or a movie, rest or even sleep. Because she enjoyed meeting new people—both patients and staff—and learning about their lives, Mom chose talking. She was curious about where they were born, how long they had lived in the area, how many children they had, and where they met their spouse. She had an endless list of questions, and could talk with anyone.

Six weeks into her treatment, Mom called me. *"I'm so lucky. I'm so much better off than many of the other patients. We live close, so it only takes your Dad ten minutes to drive me to the treatment center. I've made many new friends. The nurses are quite nice and helpful and so far I've felt pretty good."* She sounded upbeat, as usual.

I found Mom's positive attitude amazing, especially when I learned that she had been opposed to having any treatment.

Before the chemo she felt fine; in fact, she would not have known she was sick if the doctor had not told us. It was her decision whether or not to fight the cancer; if she chose no treatment, then she would live each day to the fullest until the cancer took over. Her preference was no treatment, but Dad convinced her to try chemo, hoping to prolong her life.

Mom's reaction to the chemo wasn't too bad, except she was disappointed at losing her hair. One of the nurses administering the chemotherapy suggested that we shop for a wig before all her hair fell out, which we did. I decided I would buy a wig, too; that way when we were together we could both show off our new hairdos.

A friend of Mom's told me about a specialty store in Palm Desert that sold wigs. The store was close to a Mexican restaurant that Mom and I enjoyed, so I bribed her with lunch if she would accompany me to the wig shop.

"Oh my," I exclaimed, surprised to see so many hairstyle choices waiting for us as I opened the shop door, letting Mom enter first.

"Hi. My name is Joyce," said the petite, blonde, store clerk. "Thanks for coming in. Are you interested in trying on wigs?"

"Yes we are, thank you," I replied. "My mom is receiving chemo and she's starting to lose her hair."

Joyce pulled out a chair on rollers for Mom, pointing to the vanity cabinet. "Put your purses in the unlocked bottom drawer. The key's in the lock on a pink elastic band that will fit on your wrist as you tour the store." She also handed us two cold bottles of water, requesting that we place them in the vanity cup holders, between the two mirrors. "Take your time," she said. "We like our customers to touch the hair, and pick up the Styrofoam heads. That way, they can turn them around and see both the sides and the back. Let me know which ones you want to try on," she added, "and I'll bring them to you. Also, if you choose one, we'll trim the hair to fit your face. Just take your time; we really want you to enjoy yourself."

The experience was even better than trying on shoes at our favorite store. When we looked at Mom's watch, we couldn't believe we had been there three hours; it seemed like only thirty minutes. We tried wigs with hair longer and shorter than ours, in various shades of blonde, brunette, and red, and we laughed in amazement at the way each different wig changed our looks! Yet at the end, we both selected wigs that were very similar to the color and shape of our own hair. My love for change had temporarily ceased; knowing I would be losing Mom was all the change I could handle.

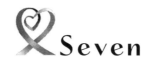

Seven

Visits to the Cemetery
February – August

Eventually I moved through the shock and fear that had accompanied the return of Mom's cancer. Even in the midst of sorrow, there were many times during the following months when our shared moments turned into fond memories, such as our visits to the cemetery.

When I flew down for Mom's first chemo treatment, she met me at the Palm Springs International Airport. Sonny Bono, the mayor of Palm Springs and one half of the Sonny and Cher singing duo, had died in a skiing accident the prior month. He was buried in Desert Memorial Park in Cathedral City, which we would pass on our drive home. As we drove closer to the cemetery, Mom and I discussed Sonny's unanticipated death.

"I feel so sorry for Sonny's family. They had no time to tell him how much they loved him and his friends had no opportunity to let him know how important he was in their life."

"Yes Mom," I said, "but on the other hand, it was instantaneous; he didn't have to suffer."

"True, but look how devastating his unexpected death was to his wife, his two young children, his mother and even to Cher."

"You know, Mom," I said, "some people die unexpectedly and quickly, and others fight off death for years. We could debate the pros and cons of dying suddenly or living with a life-limiting illness and having time to really enjoy each day and say good-bye to loved ones. But, as one of my friends might say, 'It is already written.' That decision is not ours to make."

I was driving Mom's car, and by now we were close to the cemetery. "Do you want to stop and see Sonny's grave? To pay our respects?"

"You bet I do; it'll be a new adventure. And Dad's golfing, so we don't need to rush home."

We turned left off Ramon Road onto DaVall Drive, and then took the first left into the small cemetery. Neither of us had been there before, so we weren't sure whether to turn left or right on the interior drive. It never occurred to us to stop across the street at the large mortuary to get a map, but it didn't matter. We turned right, and had no problem at all finding Sonny's grave—we just followed the crowd. It turned out that we were not the only ones who wanted to pay our respects.

Desert Memorial Park was well maintained, and we welcomed the shade from the tall trees framing both sides of the narrow two-lane road. I must admit it was awkward walking over gravestones with my mother, knowing she was battling cancer, and that an untimely death might be in her future. But it turned out to be something fun to do, and a first for us: "star hunting" at a cemetery.

Nearing the crowd, I found a space on the right, and was able to parallel park between two SUVs. We walked to the center of the crowd, to the marker showing where Sonny was buried, but his gravestone was not yet in place. Stopping for a few minutes, we talked about how hard it was to believe he was really gone. A few others had followed us, so we moved off to the side, noticing how quiet their voices became the closer they walked to his grave.

After paying our final respects to Sonny and his family, I guided Mom back to the car. We made our way along the perimeter of the cemetery, where several families were placing fresh flowers on graves. Pleased to have taken the time to stop, we headed home for lunch.

A few months later, on May 14, 1998, Frank Sinatra died. It was a dark day for Mom, who had enjoyed listening to his music and reading about his life adventures for more than forty-five years. Frank was buried at Desert Memorial Park, the same cemetery as Sonny.

When picking me up at the airport on my first visit after Sinatra's death, Mom asked if we could stop at the cemetery again, this time to see Sinatra's grave. Driving through the entrance, we looked around, and saw a group of people gathered close to the Ramon Road side of the cemetery, south of Sonny's grave. We assumed they were like us, wanting to pay respects to one of the stars of Mom's generation, and we were right. There, between the gravestones of his mother, Dolly Sinatra, and his father, Frank, we stood above the body of our beloved Frank Sinatra.

Mom and I were both teary eyed, so to give us something else to think about, I suggested we visit Sonny's grave again to see if his permanent gravestone was in place. Mom agreed, and we made our way toward his grave. As we looked at the new gravestone, we both gasped. It read:

Salvatore Phillips "Sonny" Bono

February 16, 1935
January 5, 1998

And The Beat Goes On

How fitting. We loved it. We wondered if using the title from Sonny and Cher's number-one hit song had been Sonny's prearranged request, or if the idea came from his family. It didn't matter; it was perfect.

We had fun on the ride home, each of us taking turns guessing what might be engraved on Sinatra's permanent gravestone. Perhaps it would be *Come Fly With Me*, or *Old Blue Eyes*, or *It's Now or Never*, or even *I'll Be Seeing You*. We enjoyed trying to come up with the answer, but we weren't even close.

A few months later we drove to the cemetery once more to see Sinatra's grave. Only Frank Sinatra could get Mom and me to a cemetery so close to her impending death, but we were ever so glad we made

31

the trip. Once more, we gasped with delight when we read the engraving on the permanent gravestone:

Francis Albert Sinatra

December 12, 1915
May 14, 1998

The Best Is Yet To Come

We smiled all the way home.

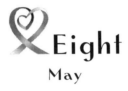

Eight

May

After three months of chemotherapy at the oncology center--enduring constant poking in her veins, multiple blood tests, daily shots for weeks at a time, and numerous trips from home to her oncologist--it was time for one more test. Mom had an MRI (short for magnetic resonance imaging), a scan that would provide her doctor with the information he needed to determine whether the tumor in her lung was growing or shrinking. Like every cancer patient undergoing treatment, she fervently hoped the results would confirm the tumors were shrinking. In order that the three of us could receive the news together, I flew down from Northern California.

A young girl in scrubs escorted us into a very small examination room. "The doctor will be with you in a minute," she said, pulling the pocket door closed.

The door made me think that the tiny room started life as a storage closet, then when the need arose it had been turned into an exam room, with its walls painted "boring beige." Two walls were covered with the obligatory medical posters, with one illustrating through a multitude of bright colors what purported to be my complex inner workings, and the other warning me of the dangers ahead should I decide to smoke, eat too much, or not exercise. Too bad the room didn't have a mirror. I wondered if Mom and I looked alike in our wigs.

Mom sat in the dark brown plastic chair. I jumped up to sit on the medical examination table, the stiff white paper wrinkling loudly. Dad leaned against the single row of cabinets, placing the *Sports Illustrated* he had picked up in the waiting room on the metal shelf.

We heard a knock on the door and turned to see the doctor, wearing a knee-length white lab coat over everyday street clothes. Dad and I shook his hand, pleased to see him give Mom a tender hello touch on her arm.

"Sorry to keep you waiting," he began, turning to Mom and getting right to the point. "Unfortunately, the tests show your tumor is growing. We can try a stronger and more expensive drug during the next three months, which might shrink the tumor, or you can stop the treatments."

I found myself gasping for air, as if his words had sucked the oxygen out of the room. The doctor didn't speak, but instead waited for one of us to break the silence.

We were too embarrassed to cry, scream, or even hug one another in front of the doctor, so we remained silent, until I asked the two questions the three of us were thinking: "Without further treatment, how much longer does she have?" And, "If she were your wife, what would you recommend?"

Turning from me to Mom, he said, "There is no easy answer. Everyone's body responds differently, and the cancer grows at different rates. We don't like to guess. But because your daughter asked, my thoughts are that you could live for anywhere from three months to a year, perhaps a little longer. If you were my wife, I would suggest ending the treatment, which should make you feel better and improve your quality of life."

I don't remember leaving that room or getting into the car, but I remember the silent ride home and changing into my jogging clothes. I wanted out of the house to give my folks time to talk and absorb the news, plus I needed exercise, to run until my heart hurt from overexertion, not from grief. That evening, after a very quiet dinner, we turned on the TV and pretended to watch the evening news, *Jeopardy*, and *Wheel of Fortune*. We sought distraction over conversation, and I went to bed early.

The next morning, Mom announced her decision—she was done with chemotherapy. In her mind she wasn't giving up, but rather acknowledging that we don't live forever. She wanted to feel better and enjoy each remaining day as best she could.

Someone should have asked me how to spell cancer, because I believe it is spelled incorrectly. Cancer is most definitely a four-letter word.

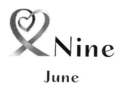

Nine

June

O ur plan was for Mom and Dad to sell their three-bedroom desert home and buy another property nearby so that after Mom passed, Dad would have a smaller, less expensive home to maintain.

Because we talked openly about Mom's impending death, we also planned for it in other ways. The three of us met with an estate-planning lawyer, who made sure that Mom and Dad's wills, revocable trusts, durable powers of attorney, and health care documents were up to date and drafted pursuant to their current wishes. We added my name to Grandma's checking account and their bank accounts, so that I could also pay bills and sign checks if the need arose. Dad made a list with the numbers of their bank accounts and retirement funds. He promised to update the list when needed, as he reminded me where it and other important documents were filed in his den.

Thank goodness my parents discussed these matters with me. Having their legal matters in order avoided a lengthy California probate. Although any death is accompanied by paperwork, at least I didn't have the added stress of legal matters to deal with during my grief.

Dad found a two-bedroom condo he liked, just a few blocks from their current house. He spent the summer downsizing and watching the cooking channel; meal preparation was becoming his job.

In packing for their move, Dad sorted through fifty-two years of memories, donating or giving away whatever they didn't want to move. Mom helped when she could, but most of the move--and by now half of the cooking--fell on Dad. He was doing too much by himself, but he didn't want to pay movers to help him. He was already pinching pennies, planning to live without Mom's Social Security and pension.

My parents loved living in the Palm Springs area. Winter days are sunny, with temperatures generally between sixty and eighty degrees, perfect for enjoying time outside. They also enjoyed the summer, even though the temperatures can be quite hot. Although their home was air conditioned, the garage was not; it might be well over one hundred degrees in there. Dad spent a lot of time that summer in the garage sorting, packing, and storing boxes.

It was no surprise when Dad started to complain. There was nothing he could pinpoint--he didn't have pain in his hip or a sore knee or back--but he didn't feel well. He refused to see a doctor, but we did notice times when he had trouble catching his breath. We assumed it was overexertion in the hot desert summer.

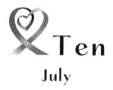

Ten

July

In July, my Aunt Doris and Uncle Charles celebrated their fiftieth wedding anniversary. Mom and Dad had stood up for Dad's sister, Doris, when she was married in 1948, and they wanted to join in the celebration. For their special occasion my Aunt and Uncle splurged, inviting close friends and family to enjoy afternoon cocktails, an early dinner, and dancing for four hours on a rented yacht, cruising through Newport Beach Harbor. I wasn't sure Mom would be up to attending, but she insisted on it. We dressed early, smiling wryly as together we donned our wigs and angel pins. I discovered that I enjoyed not having to style my hair, and also that wig hair was immune to fog damage, which for me meant no curls or frizzy hair.

That afternoon, Mom sat outside on the back of the yacht, wearing large-rimmed, dark glasses, the sun warming her body while she had the pleasure of visiting with friends she hadn't seen for years. Each time I glanced her way, she was smiling. My mom lived in the moment. She was having a good day and not thinking of the future. Remembering to live in the moment was one of the many lessons Mom taught me during the "Last Months."

My favorite memory of that day stems from watching Dad stroll to the back of the yacht to invite Mom to join him on the dance floor, just as he had done the day they met. Hand-in-hand they walked; and soon, arm-in-arm, they were swaying with the music. We all felt in our hearts it was their last dance. To the rest of the guests, it appeared that they were having fun like the others; to the three of us, that dance was the culmination of their meeting, falling in love, sharing a life and a daughter, and now acknowledging their good days were coming to an end.

Their dance would end because the music would stop.

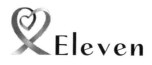

Eleven
August and September

Even though Mom wasn't feeling well, she never complained. The meds she had taken during the chemotherapy treatments had caused her to gain more than twenty pounds. The excess weight didn't show in her face, arms, or legs, but it hung around her middle, which she hid by not tucking in her colorful, loose blouses. She still looked good, and there were hours when I could deceive myself into believing maybe the doctor was wrong, that Mom wasn't dying.

In August, my parents moved into their new Palm Desert home. On one hand, the move was good in that it occupied their time and gave them something else to think about. Yet it must have been hard for Dad to be excited about the move, knowing he would soon be living there alone.

Dad still wasn't feeling well and finally agreed to see his doctor. The doctor said his blood work and X-rays were normal, so in September they decided to come north and visit me. They shared the drive with their dear friends Dave and Adele, whom they had known for over forty years. During the day, I would work at the office while the four of them would help with my household projects: hanging pictures, potting plants, and organizing my garage. My parents always wanted to help me. No matter that I was in my forties and they weren't feeling their best; I was their child, and it was their pleasure to help me in any way possible.

In July, I had rescued two twelve-week-old kittens: a calico I named Pumpkin, and her gray and white litter sister I named Mischief. They would chase each other through my condo, slide on the polished wood floors, slam against walls, and roll over each other, then get up and do it all again. After tiring themselves, they would crawl into the closest lap and sleep as deeply as they had played. The kittens helped us laugh, which lightened the mood. I have seen cards that read: "Cats are angels with fur," and for me, that was true. They brought much needed sunshine as I journeyed through that life-changing storm.

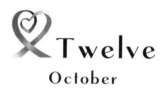

Twelve

October

I have heard that good things come in threes, and three good things happened to me that October, even though I didn't know it at the time.

The first weekend I flew south to visit my parents and enjoy the October weather, when summer temperatures start to fall, giving way to perfect desert weather. The next day, I woke up early to enjoy a morning jog and on my way to the kitchen, I was surprised to find Mom dressed and reading in the living room.

"*Care to join me for a walk?*" she asked a bit nervously.

"Of course," I smiled, wondering what was so important to interrupt her morning routine of reading the newspaper in bed with Dad. I grabbed my running cap, tied my shoelaces, and met her at the front door.

As soon as the door shut, she blurted out, "*Your Dad has stopped playing golf, isn't eating much, takes longer naps, and goes to bed early. He isn't complaining, but I'm scared something serious is wrong. You know that he loves to play golf, but he tells me he doesn't have the energy.*"

I stopped, turning to face her. "But I thought the doctor said his tests results are normal."

"Yes, but more tests are scheduled. Until they find what's wrong and get him healthy again, he isn't up to doing much."

We started walking again as I digested her news. I was deep in thought and nearly tripped over her next words.

"I want to die at home, with you taking care of me."

I could not believe my ears. My mind started racing, screaming out thoughts: I'm not a nurse, how will I take care of you? Dad will recover; why can't he take care of you? You live in Southern California yet I live in Northern California; will you move? How will I handle the emotional strain? You want to die in my home? What about my job? What about my life?

But instead of saying what I was thinking, I stopped to give her a big hug, "Yes Mom, I promise to take care of you at home until...well...I'll take care of you." I must have said those words with a confidence I didn't have, because I saw peace wash over her face before she smiled, held me close, and whispered, *"Thanks."*

Her surprise request turned out to be the first good thing to happen to me that month. To this day, I am glad she asked me to care for her. She was my best friend, yet in the process of honoring her wish, we grew even closer.

The second good thing came a week later, when I met one of our future caregivers on a hike in the Headlands, an area just north of the San Francisco Golden Gate Bridge. Carolyn, the wife of an office colleague, was extremely fit and led hikes in the area.

A friend visiting from Hawaii knew that I needed a change of pace, and she suggested we enjoy a hike. It would be a fun way to exercise, meet new friends, and walk through the hills to the coast. We were experiencing sunny October weather, and I needed a break, so we joined in the fun.

There were eight of us on the hike. Trekking through rolling hills (with occasional stunning ocean views), we took turns walking with one another, so that we might all become acquainted. Later, as I shared the day with Mom, I told her about one of the hikers named Warren, a man in his thirties. At the time Warren was close to graduating from nursing school. His dream was to help others, and he hoped to get a job at the University of San Francisco Medical Center. Mom and I were loyal Costco shoppers, and we both wore Costco socks, which are easily identifiable. Mom laughed when I added that not only would she like Warren, but also that she would identify with him, as he was the only other hiker wearing Costco socks.

Later in the month, the third gift arrived: my hearing about the benefits of hospice. By telephone, through a friend, I was introduced to Vickie. Like me, Vickie was an only child; like me, her Mom had terminal cancer, and like me, her Mom wanted to die at home, to be cared for by her husband and daughter. Vickie's Mom had died earlier in the year and her Dad had been able to take care of her Mom, with Vickie's help and the help of hospice. To this day, I have yet to meet Vickie in person, even though the information she provided helped me honor my mother's wish. Mom's doctor didn't tell us about hospice; and without Vickie's insight, I wouldn't have known where to turn.

Vickie called me on October 18. I remember the date because I saved the notes I took during her phone call. She told me that hospice provided an invaluable service during the care of her mother. My notes read as follows:

✓ Connect with hospice as soon as possible, they provide resources at every step of the way

✓ Can change team members if personality conflict

✓ Nurse provides free management and free medication

✓ The dying process is like childbirth--it is different for everyone

✓ Some stop eating

✓ Energy level starts decreasing, energy units decrease with time, to save energy units use shower chair, tray to eat, don't use energy units to do daily stuff, save for visits with friends or to watch a movie

✓ Will start sleeping more

✓ Moments of disorientation or moments of clarity. Vickie did things in her mother's room as much as possible, just to be in the room, like fold laundry or read the newspaper, whether her mother was awake or asleep

✓ Communication is very important

✓ Keep notebook by the bed to record when pain and other meds are administered

✓ Near the end her mom couldn't talk but she could hear

✓ Hospital bed good for her mom, can sit up, watch TV, doze

✓ Vickie's Dad slept in twin bed next to mom in hospital bed

✓ No regrets, no guilt, did all needed and had to do; walked away a full-grown adult

✓ Things could be worse; siblings fight

Vickie gave me examples of what to expect and warned me that caring for a dying loved one was difficult work, but very worthwhile. My notes ended with something that actor Paul Newman had said about hospice care proving that much can be done for people at the end of their lives. He affirmed that an individual's worth, dignity, and growth have no end. Paul Newman was a philanthropist and a member of the National Hospice Foundation Board of Governors. In 1988 he founded the first of several Hole-in-the-Wall Gang Camps for children with cancer and other life-limiting illnesses. Near the end of his life, after he finished chemotherapy treatment in the hospital, Newman told his family that he, too, wanted to spend the end of his life surrounded by the comforts of home. And he did.

During my next visit to Mom and Dad's, one evening was particularly difficult for Mom. Although she still didn't complain, I watched her cough up little bits of blood throughout the evening. I was scared, wondering if her time was coming to an end much faster than I was ready to accept. I raised the issue of calling hospice to help Mom. But even with Vickie's advice, I didn't know enough to answer Dad's questions. "Isn't hospice just for people with certain kinds of illnesses?" he asked. "How much does it cost?"

Unfortunately the attorney in me, factual and precise, responded, "Hospice is for anyone whose illness is known to be life-limiting and has six months or less to live." All Dad heard me say was "six months or less to live.

"Well, your mother is going to live for much longer than six months," yelled Dad. "So I don't want to discuss it any further!" Mom wouldn't disagree, and that ended the discussion.

Instead of helping, I had blown it. I was furious with myself. I should have answered differently, and I would have if I had done more research. But Dad was still the head of our family, so I dropped the subject, unaware of the turn of events that would soon cause me to learn that Vickie was right: help from the hospice experts was invaluable.

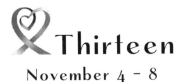

Thirteen

November 4 – 8

Mom turned seventy-five on Wednesday, November 4. That night, their friends Dave and Adele took my parents to Ruth's Chris Steak House off Highway 111 in Palm Desert to celebrate with cocktails and dinner. Seated in a booth for four, Dad and Dave shared a medium rare rib eye steak and Mom and Adele shared a medium rare filet. Each steak was served on a sizzling hot platter, smothered with melted butter and carefully placed before them with the "do not touch, this plate is hot" warning. They shared sides of potatoes au gratin, grilled mushrooms, and creamed spinach. Although they were full after a robust meal, they agreed to divide one slice of chocolate "sin" cake in honor of Mom's birthday.

I arrived in Palm Springs the following day, around one in the afternoon. My office agreed I could work from my parent's home for a week and a friend agreed to watch my kittens. I wanted to take care of Mom while Dad stayed in the hospital the next Monday, Tuesday, and Wednesday for more tests. They were still trying to determine why he felt so bad.

Before driving home to the Orange County area, Dave and Adele joined us for a late lunch at Las Casuelas in Rancho Mirage. It was a sunny, clear, warm afternoon and the lunch crowd had departed.

We sat outside on the garden patio, under the shade trees. My parents were hungry that day. They were happy I was able to help and so for a few hours that afternoon, we forgot our troubles. We sipped margaritas, munched on chips dipped in guacamole, and reminisced and laughed while enjoying a Mexican feast.

Saturday night, the three of us went to a party at the Monterey community clubhouse. Neither Mom nor Dad was feeling very well, so I drove the six blocks to the gathering. I was surprised that when they arrived at the party, they both rallied; no one would have known that either of them didn't feel well. I spent the evening watching in awe their upbeat behavior as they laughed and joked with their friends. Dad wore a soft blue sports jacket, brown slacks, slip on dress shoes, and a peach colored short sleeve shirt. Mom was wearing white slacks, low white heels, a bright green and white jacket over a navy blue blouse, with large white earrings. In my eyes my parents still made a striking couple.

That evening, before removing her make-up and crawling into bed, Mom mustered the energy to complete her evening job. Each night she would add water and grounds to the coffee pot and place the mugs on the kitchen counter. Every morning Dad would start his day by walking out of the house to the end of the driveway, picking up the *Los Angeles Times* and the *Desert Sun*, then returning to the kitchen where he would turn on the coffee maker and read the sports section while the coffee brewed. When it was ready, he would pour the coffee, tuck the newspapers under one arm, place two steaming mugs on a tray and return to their bedroom. For as long as I can recall, Mom and Dad started most days in bed, reading the newspaper, discussing current events, laughing over the comics, and sipping their morning coffee.

Sunday morning I was up before six. Sitting at their kitchen table for two, looking through the sliding door to the outside patio, I could see the sun rising over the homes across the fairway, the night sky shifting into orange and blue hues of sunrise. I had turned on my laptop; it was quiet, a good time to catch up on work.

That morning, Dad walked into the kitchen carrying the newspapers but didn't say hello as I expected. Instead he walked by me, placed the newspapers on the counter, and, with his back to me, stood in front of the kitchen sink looking out the window. At first I thought he was looking for golfers, until I noticed he was gripping the kitchen counter with both hands, holding on and squeezing so hard that his knuckles were white. I suddenly realized he was trying to catch his breath.

I whispered, "Dad, are you okay?"

"Yes, just give me a minute," he slowly replied.

In that moment I realized Dad was extremely sick. I had been so focused on Mom that I had not paid attention to Dad. It was so quiet I could almost hear my life shift, again.

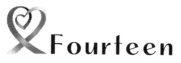

Fourteen

November 9 – 12

Monday morning I drove Mom and Dad to Eisenhower Medical Center in Rancho Mirage, a short ten-minute drive from their home. After dropping them off at the front entrance, Mom and Dad walked inside while I parked the car. Dad checked himself in and filled out all the paperwork.

We took the elevator to Dad's room on the third floor at the end of the hall, walking past the nurse's station. I was carrying a navy corduroy travel bag that Mom packed with several spy novels, Dad's razor and shaving cream, his green robe, slippers, two pair of boxers, his reading glasses and ChapStick. The room was painted a muted rose. The two windows let in light but didn't hinder his view of the suspended TV near the foot of his bed. As I left Mom alone to visit with Dad, I saw her place his reading glasses on the nightstand next to the phone. I took the elevator down to the lobby, then walked outside to participate in a work conference call. The office was busy, not the best time for me to be away. Thank goodness for cell phones, laptops, and an understanding company. Later I returned to say good-bye, then drove Mom home to rest while Dad had a few tests.

Monday night I cooked dinner for the two of us. The house was far too quiet without Dad. Mom had started taking sleeping pills before bed. Though I could have used a good night's rest, I didn't want to do the same. What if she needed me and I didn't wake up to hear her? Tuesday she awoke rested, but not me; I had tossed and turned all night. I had too many thoughts in my head. I was concerned I wouldn't have time to do all the office work that needed to be done. It hurt to think about life without Mom, and now I was frightened that Dad was also seriously ill. How could I care for both of them?

After a cup of coffee, dressed in black shorts, a black T-shirt, socks and my Nike jogging shoes, I walked outside. It felt good to stretch, breathe in the crisp morning air, and hope for a bit of tan while I jogged the short three miles to the hospital. My sports attire drew a few stares when I walked through the lobby, but soon I was alone in the elevator, moving up to the third floor. I removed my baseball cap before I entered Dad's room, pleased to find him sitting up in bed, coffee on his nightstand, reading the *Desert Sun*.

"Hi, Lumpy," he smiled. Lumpy was his term of endearment for me. He called me that when I was a wee one, with, I guess, lumps in my diaper. That term must have made him laugh, although I never found it too funny. Anyhow, that was what he called me when he was in a good mood.

"An hour ago they told me that my procedure has been moved to tomorrow morning. Will that work with your schedule?" he asked.

"Not a problem," I said. "I'll call the airline and try to move my flight back a few days."

"Wonderful," he said. "That will make your mom happy too."

We talked for about fifteen minutes. I brought him a cup of ice to chew on, made sure he didn't need anything else, then jogged home. I called Alaska Airlines and changed my flight. My whispers were telling me I should not leave Mom alone while Dad was in the hospital.

Tuesday was a good day. Mom and Dad were happy that I was staying a few more days and I was able to work the rest of the day, dropping Mom off to visit with Dad a few hours in the afternoon. I picked her up at six, and drove her to the nearby IHOP to satisfy her desire for buttermilk pancakes smothered with strawberries and whipped cream. We were both full when we got home. I relaxed in a hot lavender bath, Mom took her sleeping pill, and we were both asleep early that night.

On Wednesday I jogged to the hospital to see Dad before his procedure, but when I got to his room, they had already moved him. I ran to surgery and found him lying with bare shoulders on the gurney outside the operating room, covered from the chest down with a white blanket. He was sucking on a wet, bright green medical sponge on a stick. He looked adorable, reminding me of a little boy enjoying a lollipop. I leaned over and gave him a kiss. "Love you Dad."

"Love you too, Lumpy."

I chatted with Dad until they told me it was time to take him into surgery. I wouldn't move until the heavy metal doors shut, blocking out the stranger wheeling him into the operating room. The procedure went well and he rested the remainder of the day.

Thursday we were up early to drive to the hospital. Mom hadn't been up to visiting Dad on Wednesday, so she was eager to kiss him and hold his hand. He was grouchy; his chest hurt from the biopsy. I left them alone, and drove back to the house to work for several hours. I picked Mom up at lunchtime, giving Dad a kiss before we left him to rest.

When the phone rang Thursday afternoon, Mom was sitting in the living room, reading her book, napping off and on. I was sitting next to the kitchen phone, working on my laptop at the kitchen table. I answered because Mom had so many dear friends calling to see how she was and to ask about Dad that while she loved the calls, they were becoming physically exhausting.

It was Dad's doctor telling us that his biopsy results were in. Dad had lung cancer.

I could not believe it. I wanted to scream and throw-up at the same time. I wanted to slam down the phone and run away. I wanted to burst into tears. My head was throbbing. I prayed I was dreaming. It couldn't be that Dad also had cancer in his lungs. Was that really possible? Dad never smoked, it wasn't fair. We had enough troubles. Now Dad too had lung cancer. I wondered which one of my parents was going to die first?

Because my Mother was in the other room and could easily hear me, I tried to be calm. "Where do we go from here?" I quietly asked the doctor.

The doctor suggested strong doses of chemotherapy. He said he would release Dad to come home tomorrow and that he had already set up home health care to come and bathe and shave Dad twice a week.

The doctor had also already scheduled Dad to begin chemo at ten o'clock the following Monday. Before he hung up he asked me if I knew where the chemo treatment center was.

"Oh yes," I whispered, "only too well."

In shock, I hung up the phone. Escape was not possible. Truth was the only answer. Tears streaming down my face, I slowly walked into the living room to tell Mom--my best friend--that Dad, her best friend, also had lung cancer.

The rest of that afternoon and evening is a blur. I remember making numerous phone calls to our friends, telling them the devastating news. I remember trying to figure out how I was going to cope. I could not leave my parents alone, not now, not without finding full-time help to come in. Oh my gosh, I thought, over time that could become so expensive.

I had a sleepless night, and the next morning I started my "wear more eye make-up than usual" regime. I thought if I wore tons of eye make-up, I would keep my crying to a minimum. It turned out to work for me. As soon as I took it off at night, I would start crying, and if I was lucky, I would eventually fall asleep in my tear-soaked pillow.

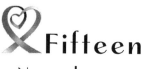

Fifteen

November 13

I learned that the human spirit is resilient. Even though I woke up to Friday the Thirteenth, I found myself thinking that if Dad had to have cancer, lung cancer wasn't that bad. I had heard of others who had lung cancer. They took chemo and they survived, so maybe Dad would be okay, but those thoughts vanished when we arrived at the hospital to bring Dad home.

Dad looked twenty years older than he had the day before. Without waiting for us, someone had told him he had lung cancer.

Now he knew why he felt so bad. He believed he had let us down because he couldn't help us with Mom's care. He was defeated, furious at his body for failing him and tired of the fight. He was wearing an oxygen hose under his nose, a new permanent fixture. He was so weak he could barely stand to move from the hospital wheelchair into our car. I knew he had lost his will to fight, perhaps to live.

When we got home, Mom and I settled him into bed. I tried to get him to eat, but he didn't have an appetite. None of us did.

Soon after we were home, a delivery man showed up with two huge metal containers of oxygen. They looked like beer kegs to me. He placed them in the hallway outside my room in front of my parents' bedroom, seemingly pleased to tell me he had brought a fifty-foot oxygen hose so that Dad could walk all over our home while connected to the tank. He then gave me what seemed to be extremely complex instructions on how to change the oxygen when the first tank ran out. Not only was I in charge of caring for Mom and Dad, I was also in charge of Dad's oxygen lifeline.

My comfort zone had disappeared. Instead of an attorney working with confidence on a transaction, I needed to be a nurse, but had no medical training. I didn't know how to make Dad comfortable, I had no idea how to deal with this recent health crisis. I was worried I would do something wrong and one of the oxygen tanks might explode. I was afraid to acknowledge that Dad was gravely ill. I was terrified of life irrevocably changing, of losing my parents. Face it, I was just plain afraid.

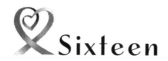

Sixteen

The Green Onion Ladies
November 14

O n Saturday morning, with Mom's help, Dad took off his pajamas and put on slacks and a golf shirt. He wanted to sit in the living room. One week before, he could walk from their bedroom to the living room in less than ten seconds. Saturday it took him five minutes to walk that distance. Leaning on me, he would take a short step, stop to catch his breath, pull the oxygen hose behind him, and repeat the process. Slowly he made his way to sit in Mom's swivel chair, where through the sliding window he could watch the golfers on the fairway outside their back patio. Those happy, laughing golfers were living the life my Dad had once enjoyed. Dad looked so dejected and sad, sitting with his shoulders slumped, tethered to the oxygen, silent in his thoughts. He hadn't been in the living room more than fifteen minutes when he asked me to help him back to his bedroom. He didn't want to watch the golfers nor did he want to talk to his friends.

We were a family without an appetite. Fortunately, throughout his life, Dad had enjoyed eating three meals a day. Old habits are hard to break and his was no exception. That Saturday morning, Dad asked me what I was fixing for dinner.

"What do you want?" I asked.

"What food do we have in the house?"

"I can drive to the grocery store and buy anything you want. Mom, what do you feel like eating?"

"I don't care, whatever your Dad wants."

This went on for ten minutes until we finally decided on a roasted chicken with mashed potatoes, which required a trip to the store.

The grocery store became my "stress free" zone. I didn't feel guilty leaving Mom and Dad alone in the house because I had a valid reason to be out--I was buying needed groceries. I carried my cell phone, but only in case they needed to reach me; otherwise, I didn't answer calls. I parked the car in the empty rows away from the store, buying myself thirty seconds of fresh air. Even though I only needed a few items, I took my time. I strolled up and down each aisle, acting as though I was searching for products, wondering if my heartache was visible.

In the cookie aisle I watched a young mother with her two teenage children, buying for a field trip. In the produce section I glanced at a lady buying sweet corn on the cob. Would her family laugh during dinner conversation tonight? I lingered next to a man buying cabernet. Would he be giving that to the host of a dinner party this evening?

Why couldn't they see that I was in a crisis? How was it that my life was crumbling but others going about their happy day? It sounds silly, but the grocery store was my reminder that one day my life would not be so crazy, sad, and full of stress. For me, the future would arrive, and I would be the one buying champagne to celebrate a happy occasion.

While in my daze the clerk handed me two plastic bags, "Would you like help to your car m'am?"

"No thank you," I said, thinking how greatly I really did need help.

I wanted so much to do everything possible to make Mom and Dad happy. If I could take away their suffering for just a few minutes, I felt good. So that night I was especially conscientious with the dinner preparations, wanting the meal to be perfect. The chicken was in the roasting pan; the potatoes had been peeled, sliced, and were boiling in lightly salted water; the salad was made; dinner rolls were ready to go in the oven; and I had set a lovely table, with a gold tablecloth and a vase of fresh white carnations.

When I walked into their bedroom to tell them dinner would be ready in about thirty minutes, Dad said, "You bought green onions for dinner, didn't you?"

"Of course," I lied.

Darn it! I wanted this meal to be perfect, but because I didn't eat green onions, I hadn't thought to buy them. I am not prone to lying, but these were desperate times and that lie just slipped out. Now that I had said I had green onions, I couldn't drive to the store to buy them. What was I going to do?

I walked back to the kitchen and called their neighbor Gen to see if she had any. Gen knew how sick both Mom and Dad were and she understood that I wanted to make them happy in any way I could—hence the urgency of my green onion quest. Gen didn't have any, but she said she would make some calls to see if any of the neighbors did.

I smile as I think how many calls were made that evening for such a seemingly small but meaningful request.

"Karen, it's Gen. Do you have any green onions?"

"No, but last week I ate at Jane's, and she served green onions with lunch."

"Thanks, I'll try Jane."

"Jane, its Gen. Do you have any green onions?"

"No, but I know that Jack, Fran's husband, likes green onions."

"Okay, thanks."

The calls went round the neighborhood in a desperate search.

Fifteen minutes later the phone rang. It was a neighbor who lived four blocks away. "I have green onions," were her only words.

"Meet you in front of the house in five minutes," I said.

"Dad, I'm going outside to put the trash cans out," I yelled into their bedroom. "I'll be right back."

It was dark outside when the neighbor drove by and handed me a bag of green onions.

"Thanks so much," I said.

She smiled and drove away in the night. I chuckled to myself, feeling like a character in a novel that had just completed an illegal drug deal.

I shoved the bag under my sweater and smuggled it into the kitchen. Success! I was so happy.

I cut and cleaned the green onions, placed them in a glass dish on the table, and then brought out the rest of the meal. I waited with pride as together Mom and Dad very slowly walked the short distance from their bedroom to the dining table.

Dad started to gag the minute he turned into the dining area. It was the pungent smell of the green onions! Dad's body could no longer handle strong odors. "Get those green onions out of here!" he yelled.

And, just like that, there went my few minutes of happiness.

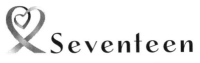

Seventeen
November 15 and 16

Sunday was a bad day. Dad felt much worse. He had no energy and was too weak to get out of bed. Walking the ten yards from his side of the bed to their bathroom was a struggle. On the plus side, so long as Dad was sitting in the bed, he was able to enjoy TV and could read the newspaper. But movement of any kind would cause him to lose his breath and leave him extremely exhausted. He didn't want to leave the house on Monday; he didn't want chemotherapy.

Monday morning I called the oncologist's office. "I need to speak to someone about my father's chemo appointment this morning."

"I can help you," the receptionist offered. "What do you need?"

"Well," I explained, "my father has a ten o'clock appointment, but he's so weak that I don't think I can get him into the car. I also don't think he can survive a rigorous chemotherapy treatment."

"No problem," she replied. "I'll cancel his chemo appointment, and you can call us back when he's ready to start."

"Wait, don't hang up," I said. "I don't know what to do. My dad is very ill. Can someone come out here to see him?" I begged.

"I'm afraid not," she said. "We just don't make house calls. But, if you want, we can make room to see him this afternoon at four."

"But I can't get him into the car. He's too weak to leave the house. What should I do?" I pleaded. "I'm not a nurse, and I don't know what to do."

"I'm sorry," she said, "but we really can't help you any further. When he gets stronger, call us and we'll schedule the chemo."

I could hear the other line ringing on her phone, so I said good-bye, hung up the receiver, put my head in my hands, and sobbed. Mom was dying, and Dad was very sick; maybe he was dying too. To make matters worse, I didn't live in the area, and I had no idea who to call for help. I was heartbroken and frustrated. I couldn't find anyone to help us.

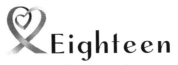

Eighteen
Finding Help
November 17

E arly Tuesday morning I walked outside to pick up the newspapers. Dad's job had now become my responsibility. I took a minute and stood still, gazing up at the stars lingering in the early morning sky. Life seemed so peaceful and orderly outside — unlike the downward spiral inside.

Later that morning, after hearing Mom and Dad talking, I walked into their room to hand them the newspapers. When I brought them coffee a few minutes later, they were both sitting up in bed reading. Looking at them, it was hard to believe that our life was upside down. They looked exactly as they had every morning of their married life, reading the newspaper together and enjoying their morning coffee before starting their day. But my broken heart told me otherwise.

I had planned to fly home later in the day, but once again my inner voice said no. Even though it would be nice to have a change of clothes (and I wanted to hold my kittens), my heart knew it was not time to leave. Both Mom and Dad looked so relieved when I told them I was going to stay for a few more days.

There were more calls to the airline, and then to the office. Everyone was very understanding. They knew I was working as much as I could; my colleague, Dick, and the rest of the legal department stepped in to handle the work I didn't have time to do. The gal watching my kittens said they were fine, and that she would continue to care for them.

By noon on Tuesday I had a throbbing headache—the worst of my life—and I thought I might soon be violently ill. I would be totally useless if that happened. I was at the end of my rope, and I needed help—but there was none.

By two that afternoon I'd had enough. Just sitting in bed, even with the oxygen, Dad was having trouble breathing, and Mom looked so sad. I had to do something.

Weeks earlier, at my request, a nurse in Mom's doctor's office had given me the phone number for a local hospice, so I decided to call. It was the only hope I had. That one call turned out to be the best phone call I ever made.

My heart was racing as I punched in the numbers. I remembered our last conversation regarding hospice. How ironic for me to be calling to help Dad and not Mom. I hated to acknowledge that he might have less than six months to live, but it could be true. I had no other options, no place else to turn.

I called the Palm Desert office of the Visiting Nurse Association of the Inland Counties, nearly in tears by the time I was transferred to a lady who listened to my story. She was soft-spoken and yet strong at the same time. During our talk I started to calm down. She asked me questions about Mom and Dad, and then she asked for our address, informing me that a nurse would be arriving at our house in the next few hours.

I hung up the phone and cried with relief. I couldn't believe that a medical professional was coming to our house. Someone would tell me how to make Dad more comfortable. Finally, help was coming.

I said a prayer of gratitude. Then I went into Mom and Dad's bedroom and asked Mom if she would mind coming into the living room.

"Mom, I called hospice, and they're sending a nurse over here in a few hours to examine Dad. Maybe they can make him comfortable."

"A nurse is coming here? We don't have to take your Father anywhere?"

"Yes, a nurse is coming here. Isn't that wonderful?"

We hugged each other in delight, extremely grateful that help was on its way. My headache was slowly receding. Someone cared about us.

Nineteen

A t 4 p.m. that afternoon the doorbell rang. Mom was sitting in the bedroom with Dad, but she quickly came into the living room. Dad stayed in bed, watching TV and resting.

I opened the front door, not knowing what to expect, simply filled with gratitude that a nurse was here to help us.

Standing before me was a lady who looked to be in her mid fifties, about five-feet tall, with short gray hair. She had the most pleasant, calming voice. "Hello, I'm Dorothy," she smiled. "I'm a nurse with the Visiting Nurse Association."

"Yes, please come in," I said. "Thanks so much for coming so quickly." Then, all in one breath, I blurted out, "I'm Rae Ann, and this is my mom, Anne. My apologies if I called you too soon, but my father, Ray, seems to be quite ill. And we know my Mom is dying, and I just don't know where else to turn or how to make Dad comfortable."

Dorothy smiled. "It's my pleasure to be here," she replied, as she walked into our house. "If you don't mind, may I speak with you and your Mother before I talk with your Father? I'd like to explain our service to both of you. Then, if you agree, I'll speak with your Dad. Is that okay?"

"Yes," I replied, as Dorothy followed me into the living room. "And thank you again. I hope I didn't call too soon," I said. "And I really hope this isn't a wasted trip for you, but I didn't know where else to turn."

Dorothy sat next to me on the living room couch. Mom was close by, her swivel chair turned in our direction. Dorothy had brought a packet of information with her, along with what appeared to be a medical bag, and she listened attentively as we told her our history. We explained that Mom's cancer had returned, that it was in her lungs, and that her condition was terminal. We also told her that I was an only child, and that Mom and Dad had been married for over fifty-two years. We told her about Dad's illness, how he hadn't felt well for months, and that last Thursday we had learned he had lung cancer. We told her he was scheduled for chemo yesterday, but was too weak to leave the house.

Dorothy asked us questions about Dad. She wanted to know the names of his doctors, whether he was taking medications, and, if so, the names and dosages. She also asked for his Social Security number and whether he had supplemental health insurance. Did they have prearranged funeral plans? Mom told her they did, and gave her the information. As Mom talked, Dorothy made notes and filled out forms.

Dorothy explained that later, after she examined Dad, she would call a pharmacy to order any medication he might need. It would be delivered to our front door later in the day. Mom and I were amazed.

Dorothy asked if we needed a wheelchair, believing she could have one delivered to our house that day. She also suggested it might be easier for Dad if he rode in the wheelchair instead of walking around the house. Mom and I said yes, not seeing any downside except for the expense.

She asked if we wanted a hospital bed for Dad, explaining that she thought he might be more comfortable in a bed with a back that could be adjusted to help him sit up. That, too, could be delivered to our house that day if we wanted. Mom and I looked at each other, wondering how much this quick and effective care cost. I suggested that Dorothy ask Dad if he wanted a hospital bed.

"Okay," she said. Do you have any questions for me?"

"*If my husband agrees to hospice care, will he get to stay here at home? He won't have to go to the hospital or a nursing home, will he? And will you be our hospice nurse?*"

"Our goal," said Dorothy, "is to help you care for your husband here, in your home. I don't know who will be your hospice nurse; I'm just the nurse on call today. I may be your assigned nurse but we won't know until tomorrow when one of our social workers will come here to talk with you to determine what other ways we may help you. Oh, and if you would like a chaplain for your husband or for you, we'll make arrangements for one to come to your home. Our goal is to make sure your husband is comfortable and to give you support. We want to be sure your husband is not in pain, and we want him to live each day as best he can."

I felt comforted yet had one final question. "How much will all this hospice service cost us?"

"Since your father is eligible for Medicare," Dorothy said, "our service won't cost you anything. Hospice is a federally sponsored government program, and the service is covered by Medicare."

"What about the cost for the medicine and the wheelchair that you said will be delivered to our home today?"

Dorothy smiled. "Everything is covered by Medicare. You don't have to pay for anything. You'll be the caregiver for your father, but we will visit, support your father, your mother, and you, and we will explain what you need to do to keep your father comfortable. Now, may I talk to your dad?"

Mom and I were amazed. We both thought this sounded too good to be true. Why hadn't someone told us about this earlier?

I led Dorothy into the bedroom, introduced her to Dad, and asked him if he would talk with her. Then, leaving the two of them together, I closed the bedroom door to give them privacy.

Mom and I were both anxious. On one hand, we were extremely relieved to know that soon Dad would be more comfortable; it was a gift to know we now had a nurse we could rely on. However, we were also scared that Dad might refuse the service. He might be mad at me for calling hospice. While the three of us had communicated very well about the fact that Mom was dying, we had not had the same conversation about Dad's condition. We were still in shock from learning he had lung cancer.

Dorothy talked with Dad for about twenty minutes. After leaving the bedroom she stopped in my bathroom to wash her hands, then walked back into the living room, telling us that Dad had agreed to be placed on hospice. We were so relieved!

Dorothy called in a prescription, explaining that it would ease Dad's pain and help him relax. We were surprised to hear that Dad was in pain, and welcomed anything that would bring him relief. She told me to start giving Dad the medication as soon as it arrived later that evening.

Dorothy said Dad didn't want a hospital bed yet. She ordered the wheelchair and a portable commode, telling us to place it next to the bed when it arrived. That way, Dad would not have to struggle and shuffle to the bathroom. I had no idea such things existed, but it sounded like a good idea to me.

Finally, Dorothy told us a little about her conversation with Dad. He had questioned her about his condition.

"I'm dying, aren't I?" he asked.

"Yes, you are," Dorothy replied softly. "We just don't know when."

"Who will take care of my wife?"

"We will," Dorothy replied.

After hearing those words, Dad shut his eyes and leaned back to rest his head on his pillow.

Dorothy had a way of calming each of us. She was in charge, but in a soft, loving way. I hated to see her leave, yet glancing at the clock I was surprised to see that she had been with us for two-and-a-half hours. While she was in the house I felt a peace I hadn't known for weeks.

Before she left, Dorothy handed me a bright pink sticker with a phone number for hospice. She suggested I place it on our telephone so I wouldn't lose it. She told me I could call the number any time, day or night, if I had questions or needed help. A hospice nurse was always available.

Dorothy left about six-thirty that evening. Both Mom and I gave her a heartfelt hug before she left and thanked her for coming to help us.

Within the hour, true to Dorothy's word, a wheelchair and a portable commode were delivered to the house. The medicine was delivered to our front door soon thereafter. Mom and I continued to be amazed. I don't know how much we really retained of what Dorothy had told us about hospice, but actions speak louder than words, and we knew instinctively that calling hospice had been the correct course of action.

♡ Twenty

Throughout that night, I got up every two hours to give Dad his medicine. Each time I walked into their bedroom to wake him, Mom was awake.

At about two in the morning, Mom was still awake, so I asked if she wanted to lie in bed with me. I know she had mixed emotions; it would be the first time in her fifty-two years of married life that she would willingly leave their bed. Yet she was forever a mom, and she could also see that I needed her. She looked at Dad, who was sleeping, and with a loving gesture she tucked the covers around him, and then walked with me back to my room.

I was sleeping in a pull-down Murphy bed in their small den. The room shared a wall with their bedroom and another wall with the hall to the living room, where the large oxygen containers were placed. We could hear the oxygen's steady gurgling sound, interspersed with Dad's irregular and extremely raspy, labored breathing.

As we lay in bed together, we whispered so as not to wake up Dad. Under different circumstances, it could have been a fun slumber party. We agreed it would be okay if we each prayed that God could take Dad if it was his time to leave us.

At 4 a.m. it was time for me to give Dad another pill. We both walked quietly into the bedroom.

"Dad, wake up. It's time for your pill," I whispered. Then again, a little louder, "Dad, open up."

"Like a bird?" Dad muttered in his sleepy state.

Mom and I giggled. "Yes," I said, "like a bird."

Dad opened his mouth and swallowed the pill. He was soon fast asleep. Yet still the deep, raspy, erratic breathing continued. Mom and I went back to my bed, said more prayers, and finally fell asleep.

Something woke us up at 6 a.m. We jumped out of bed to check on Dad and to our surprise, he was trying to stand up. We arrived by his side just in time to hold him and place him back in bed. We adjusted his covers, hoping he was comfortable, and together stood looking at him in the morning quiet.

"Honey, I can't go back to sleep. Do you mind watching over Dad while I freshen up in the shower?"

"Sure," I said. "I'll sit with him."

I sat on the edge of the bed, next to Dad. He was lying on his back. His right hand was tucked behind his head, with his left arm at his side, next to me. I held his free hand, watching him while he slept. I hated to see him suffer. For a moment I pretended he was fine, just resting peacefully, and would soon wake up to enjoy another day. I wanted more time with him, maybe one year, or just one month, or one more day. I wanted life to return to the way it used to be, when the three of us were healthy and happy. I wanted to run away and hide. I wanted my heart to stop hurting.

But most of all, I didn't want my father to suffer anymore.

77

So, between the tears, I looked down at him and said, "I love you Dad. Thank you for my life. I won't let you down. I promise I'll take care of Mom." And I prayed that if it was his time, he could go.

I was still holding his hand, wrapped up in my thoughts, when suddenly I noticed he wasn't breathing. I didn't know what to do. About that time Mom came out of the shower with a bath towel wrapped around her. To this day I believe Dad could hear us talking. I believe he heard his wife say she was going to take a shower, so he knew she would be out of the room. I believe he heard me tell him that I would take care of Mom. I believe he wanted to leave before Mom came back into the room.

"Mom, I think Dad has gone."

"What? Are you sure?"

"I don't know for sure, but I think so."

I had never seen a dead person before. I tried to feel for a pulse, but I was shaking and couldn't remember where I was supposed to touch. I remembered TV shows and thought about getting a mirror to see if there was any breath or fog on the mirror, but that seemed disrespectful.

The truth was, I knew Dad was gone because of the way he looked. I don't know how to explain it. He looked exactly the same—but entirely different. It dawned on me that his spirit had left his physical body. That was how I knew he had died.

Dad's death was nothing like what I'd seen in the movies. There was no last gasp of air, no eyes wide open; his death was serene and simple. One second he was with me, and the next he had quietly slipped away and was gone. In that extremely sacred moment, our prayers that his suffering would end had been answered.

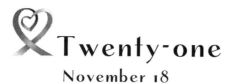

Twenty-one
November 18

O nce again, we found ourselves in uncharted territory. We didn't know what to do, so I called hospice.

Dorothy had said I could call any time, day or night. We'll see if anyone really answers that phone, I thought. It was only six-twenty in the morning, but the answering service picked up on the second ring. I told the receptionist that I needed to speak to the nurse, and I told her why. I held on while she transferred my call.

I soon heard, "Hello, this is Dorothy."

I could not believe our good fortune! Our angels were still with us.

I quickly told Dorothy what had happened. She said she would be over as soon as she could get dressed and drive to our home. She asked me if we wanted a chaplain. I hadn't thought about it and wondered how long it would take her to find one. It was a wonderful suggestion that I gratefully accepted.

Numb, and in shock, Mom and I sat in the living room and waited. Somehow we lived through our first thirty-five minutes without Dad.

Our doorbell rang just before seven that morning. Standing at our front door were Dorothy and a man she introduced as Reverend Al. I couldn't believe she had already found a chaplain. Reverend Al was a tall, big man, nearly six foot six. Neither he nor Dorothy looked or acted like they had been rushed to start their day.

"Come in, please," I said. Dorothy hugged Mom and then me. We felt as though we had known her for years. It was hard to believe our introduction had occurred only fifteen hours earlier. Dorothy went in to see Dad while we hugged and then talked with Reverend Al.

Reverend Al asked Mom, "Would you be more comfortable saying a prayer in the bedroom next to your husband?"

"Yes, please."

Dorothy, Reverend Al, Mom, and I stood next to Dad's side of the bed. The four of us held hands, forming a small circle. We prayed with Reverend Al, who had brought a small vial filed with holy water, along with a small wooden cross. He anointed Dad with the water and after our private ceremony, he handed me the cross.

At that moment, it almost seemed natural to be standing in my parents' bedroom, with a man of the cloth, saying good-bye to my father. Our small informal service provided the closure we needed.

I still have that small wooden cross. For years I stored it in the pocket of a dress jacket that I seldom wore. When I did, I would gasp in joyous surprise when my right hand, expecting an empty pocket, would touch that small wooden cross. Today the cross is in my nightstand. I will cherish it forever.

After the ceremony, Dorothy and Reverend Al left us with Dad. I said good-bye first, then left Mom to say her good-byes. I called Gen, our closest neighbor, to tell her Dad had left us, and that I would appreciate her coming over to talk with Mom while I started making the many phone calls that must be made after someone dies.

To my surprise, during the rest of the day, a steady stream of Mom's friends, including the Green Onion Ladies, came by, one at a time, to be with her.

The day was sunny and warm, perfect for Mom to sit on the back patio, under the shade of the umbrella, while friends came by to pay their respects and to give her their love. Between phone calls to family, friends, the Social Security Administration, work, and the airline, I would glance her way. I thought I knew Mom, but that day I learned even more.

Watching her hold court, I realized that she was the strong one in our family. She understood and accepted the good and bad of life. On the worst day of her life, she was able to appreciate her friends, find a reason to smile, and continue to live in the moment.

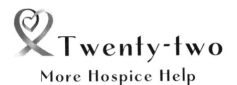

Twenty-two
More Hospice Help

That same day, while I made phone calls and Mom grieved with friends outside, Dorothy quietly handled other matters. She made arrangements for the funeral home to pick up Dad's body and dressed him in attire appropriate for his next trip.

Dorothy explained that the funeral home would certify death certificates. She told us that banks, pension plans, and insurance companies would most likely request an original death certificate. She asked me how many we would want, but I had no idea, having never seen, much less thought about a death certificate. Dorothy suggested we ask for eight originals. If we needed more we could order them later. She also collected the medicine she had ordered the night before for Dad. She counted each pill, recorded the information in a logbook, and then disposed of the remainder.

Dorothy suggested I call the Social Security office to advise them of Dad's death. She explained that was necessary so Dad's payments would be stopped. She knew Dad was a veteran and told me about a benefit due to surviving widows.

Dorothy stayed with us several hours that morning. She would make phone calls, then go sit with Mom for a while, then talk to me. Once again, she became our calming force in a sea of chaos. At one point she asked me what I was going to do about Mom.

"I plan to return to work on November 30th," I explained. "I'll have been away from the office for nearly a month, and I need to get back to work and to my home. I hope Mom will agree to come back with me, and maybe stay through the end of the year. I can't think any further than year-end. I guess when we get there, we'll revisit where we are."

Dorothy agreed with me.

During the morning, someone came in and removed the oxygen, the commode, and the wheelchair; I'm sure Dorothy had arranged for it. She also changed the sheets on Mom and Dad's bed. Before she left, Mom and I had decided that we would hold Dad's memorial service the following Tuesday. I invited Dorothy, and asked if she would bring Reverend Al. She graciously agreed. Before saying good-bye, I told her that I believed she was a gift to us from God. She smiled and replied, "Dorothy means a gift from God."

That was apparent. I knew it in my heart.

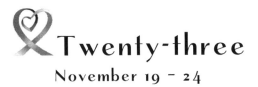

Twenty-three

November 19 – 24

I don't recall too many specifics of the next few days, but I know I spent hours talking on the phone. Mom read through every page in their address book. She wrote down the names and phone numbers of everyone she wanted me to call to invite to the memorial. Many had no idea Dad was ill and were shocked by my call. I believe, hearing the unsteady nature of my voice, most thought I was calling to tell them Mom had died.

I remember sitting with Mom at the dining table, writing Dad's obituary. Since then, I have thought about teaching an obituary writing class to make the writing easier for others. I would start by encouraging the class to talk with their parents, and to keep a list of the life events their parents would choose to highlight (for us, that door was closed). I would hand out samples of obituaries; my class would not have to read through teary eyes the obits in that morning's newspaper to become familiar with what is supposed to be covered. I would explain the cost, it's based on the number of words. When I learned this, I attacked our draft in the same way I revise a legal document, striking large portions of text. Except this was no legal document; it was the last widely distributed tribute to my Dad and I wanted it to be perfect. My class would walk out the door having learned that advance planning for an obituary would reduce stress and ensure their loved one's tribute would be of the highest quality.

Not surprisingly, the Green Onion Ladies volunteered to help. They handled all the arrangements for the memorial service, including reserving a room in the community clubhouse. They arranged the seating, podium, food, drinks, parking, and all other details. They were my lifesavers.

All Mom and I had to do was show up, which on its own was so very difficult for me. Remarkably, by the day of Dad's memorial, Mom looked very pretty and, to the untrained eye, healthy. Her wig selection had been a good choice, and she was now quite comfortable wearing it.

I had asked Mom if I could give Dad's eulogy, and she agreed (perhaps my obituary writing class might include a section on eulogies, something else I never thought about until it was too late).

I walked to the podium, and on behalf of Mom and me, I thanked everyone for attending. The small room was crowded with nearly eighty family members and friends. Looking out, I was surprised to recognize a few faces I hadn't seen for more than twenty years.

I also wore my wig—anything to make Mom feel comfortable. I had made notes of things I wanted to say, but I couldn't read them through my tears. I don't recall what I said, but I remember hearing people laugh and seeing some cry, confirming that my words conveyed my feelings. I know I thanked Dorothy, Reverend Al, and hospice for their help during our most difficult time.

That thirty minutes at the podium was the only time I ever thought that perhaps I could have been an actress, because acting was the only way I survived. I might have been teary, and I might have paused to compose myself, but I did not break down and sob, even though that is what my heart and mind wanted to do. While honoring my father, I was also saying good-bye to my mother. The hardest part was trying to follow her example: to live in the moment, putting aside the pain of yesterday, and not thinking about what tomorrow would hold. Surely living through that day gave me the strength and courage to move through the months ahead.

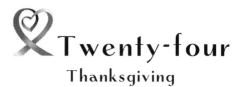

Twenty-four
Thanksgiving

Dad's memorial service was held two days before Thanksgiving. You might think it was difficult to find something to be thankful for, but it really wasn't. Mom and I were grateful to have each other, grateful that Dad was no longer suffering, and extremely grateful for the invaluable help we had received from hospice and Mom's friends.

In years past, we celebrated Thanksgiving with Aunt Doris and her family. Though we could list things to be thankful for, we weren't in the mood to celebrate, and I wasn't in the mood to cook, so we ate our Thanksgiving dinner at a resort hotel.

It was different eating our big meal in a fancy hotel, but then again, it was also different eating without Dad.

Twenty-five
November 27 - 28

Mom had a difficult decision to make. She could fly home and stay with me through the end of the year or she could continue to live by herself in the desert. She knew I had to get back to the office, and that I didn't want her to be alone. She wasn't eager to leave her home, her mother, or her friends, but with Dad gone, she decided that a change of scenery and staying with me would be her preference.

We knew her health was declining, but we didn't know how quickly. Instead of thinking she was leaving forever, it was much easier on both of us to consider her time in my home as a month's vacation. She would return to the desert in January. She loved winters in the desert when by noon she would sit on the patio, enjoying temperatures in the mid-sixties, without the need for her jacket. A tall glass of sun-brewed iced tea, the current *Good Housekeeping*, *People*, and *Sunset* magazines close at hand, and the breathtaking views of snow-covered Mount San Jacinto framed by a clear blue sky, they were paradise to Mom. Yet she knew better than to sit outside after four. Once the sun set behind the mountain the temperatures dropped quickly, then it was the perfect time to warm her feet in the living room near the fireplace. Yes, she would be ready to return in

January, but staying with me awhile was the best choice.

We spent Friday and Saturday calling her friends to tell them of her plans and to give them my address and phone number. We placed a vacation hold on the newspapers, forwarded the mail, cleaned out the refrigerator, and made sure two of the Green Onion Ladies had keys to the house and to the car we were leaving parked in the locked garage.

Next we turned our attention to ninety-six year old Grandma, who had been residing in an assisted living home for more than five years. By now, Mom knew most of the friendly staff, having become particularly well acquainted with the social director.

The assisted living staff and Dad had called her Christine, but she was always Grandma to me. After her mother died in childbirth, her father, a butcher who worked long hours, left her to be raised by a crazy stepmother, who viewed her new husband's daughter as a threat. Grandma rarely talked about those horrible years without siblings, when unbeknownst to her father, each loving hug he gave her resulted in her sitting alone for hours in a locked closet. Marrying my Grandpa was her ticket out of that house.

Mom was born in 1923 in Muskogee, Oklahoma. Her parents moved to California when she was two, yet she was always proud to be an *"Okie from Muskogee."* Grandpa came to California seeking a better life, working for his older brother selling ice cream. Soon thereafter, his brother decided they could make more money selling shoes, so Grandpa went along, but that didn't work out. Through the years, he struggled to make ends meet and frequently changed jobs. Eventually he found employment working the night shift in the Huntington Beach Oil Fields. By the time her parents settled in Huntington Beach, Mom, then in the eighth grade, had moved thirty-three times.

In the early 1950s, Grandpa was hired to manage the Huntington Beach City trailer park, located on the ocean side of Pacific Coast Highway, south of the Huntington Beach Pier. I have fond memories of staying in Grandma and Grandpa's rented house on the sand behind the life guard station with the big number "7" painted on its side. That trailer park was closed years ago, the area paved, and today is a city parking lot for beachgoers.

Being the trailer park manager, Grandpa was on call year round, with two exceptions. Every June, he and Grandma would take me to Disneyland, arriving when the gates opened and leaving only after the stunning evening fireworks display. Later in the fall they would drive to Las Vegas, always staying at the Stardust Hotel, which, when it opened in the fall of 1958, was the biggest casino in Nevada and had the largest swimming pool.

Grandpa was proud of his first and only new car, purchased when he was fifty-eight. Before he would open the driver's door of his turquoise and white, two-door hardtop, 1955 Chevrolet Bel Air, Grandpa would extinguish his cigarette, remove his ever-present black felt fedora hat with the distinctive pinched-front, adjust his bolo string tie, and make sure Grandma was settled in the car. Early on, he and Grandma struck a deal; he could smoke as many Marlboro cigarettes as he wanted, as long as he didn't smoke inside their house or car. They were married over fifty years, and he kept his end of the bargain, right up until he died in the middle of the night from lung cancer. Unfortunately my family did not know the seriousness of his illness, and he died alone in the hospital at age seventy-nine.

We wondered how Grandma would fare after Grandpa died, especially since she never learned to drive a car. At that time, they were retired and living in Leisure World, a retirement community in the city of Seal Beach, close to Mom and Dad's home in Long Beach. Grandma managed just fine, never complaining; and for the next ten years she seemed content to walk to her hair appointments, the bank, and the grocery store, with occasional visits from Mom and me.

Grandma never drank anything stronger than bottled Coca Cola, never wore slacks until she was in her eighties, and never purchased a ready-made pie. I have tried, but it is impossible to recreate her Sunday suppers. I could cut her roast beef with a fork. When no one was looking my way, I would dip the roast beef deep into the mashed potatoes and savory dark brown gravy. She used to serve thick homemade chocolate malts—until the day I distracted her, and she turned the blender on high, forgetting the lid was still on the counter. What a mess! I remember her laughing as she balanced herself against the white

Formica counter, stretching on her tiptoes to wipe the dripping chocolate ice cream off the ceiling. Thereafter, our Sunday dessert was homemade lemon pie, covered with stiff white meringue with lightly browned peaks. Everything about Grandma was good.

After my parents moved to the desert, they would frequently make the five-hour round-trip drive to Seal Beach, pick up Grandma and bring her back with them to stay for a few weeks at a time. But like many dementia sufferers, as her short and long-term memory started to disappear, the memories that remained became her reality. I recall Mom telling me about the morning she awoke at six-thirty to find Grandma sitting in their living room, wearing a pretty dress with purse in hand. Mom asked where she was going and Grandma, somewhat irritated, replied, "I am waiting for the bus to pick me up and take me to Las Vegas, don't you remember?"

Eventually it became clear that Grandma would be better off in an assisted living community where she would receive the additional care she needed. I thought her assisted living home was cozy. It wasn't the most expensive in the area, but it wasn't free either. Each resident lived in his or her own one or two-room unit. After her house was sold, we moved Grandma's double bed, nightstands, mirror, bedroom dresser, couch, coffee table, and television into her one room unit, which had a sliding glass door that opened onto a small patio off the living room area. We hung a few of her favorite framed pictures, making her large room--including its small kitchenette and bathroom with a shower--seem somewhat like home.

If I showed up unannounced, I would usually find her sitting on the couch, examining two or three of the sixty pictures she stored in a memory box on her coffee table.

"Hi Doll!" she would exclaim, breaking into a huge smile. It didn't matter if I had seen her the day before or if I hadn't visited for months, her warm greeting was always filled with love.

Before November, Mom had been able to visit Grandma several times a week. The two-and-a-half mile drive didn't take Mom more than five minutes, even if she hit every red light. But November had been a different story. We hadn't seen Grandma for a few weeks, so we hadn't told her about Dad. We had agreed her attending Dad's memorial would have been distracting to us and of no benefit to her. Now both Mom and I were heading back north. We hated to leave Grandma and spent several days discussing our options.

"Mom," I said, "if we leave Grandma here, we know she'll be well cared for, and we can call to check on her." I further explained that if we moved her to another facility near my home so that we could see her more often, we would need to research the facilities in the area, determine which had openings, choose the best one she could afford, and pay to move her furniture. I'd have to then drive down, pick her up, and hope she could handle the drive back. What was worse, we didn't know how she would adapt to the change and moving her would be costly and time consuming, unless we moved her into my house. But since I only had two bedrooms, she would have to share a room with one of us. Mom would have to watch her when I was at the office. In all honesty, we didn't need the added stress of caring for her right then. We ultimately agreed not moving Grandma would be the best for all concerned.

Late Saturday afternoon, I drove Mom to see Grandma. Upon entering the facility, we saw her sitting between two other residents, on the flowered couch in the living area, being entertained by a local pianist. We learned that his tribute to Leonard Bernstein would be over in ten minutes, which gave us time to tell Sally, the social director, where Mom would be staying and how to contact us. After the music stopped, Grandma saw us leaning against the check-in counter. "Hi Doll!" she cried out, struggling to get up from the couch.

I ran over to her, hugging her tight and kissing her cheek, content to inhale her familiar scent. By the time Mom and Grandma hugged, I had sat down and was ready to support Mom as she told Grandma our plans.

"Mom, why don't we sit here for a few minutes, do you mind?" she asked, patting the cushion beside her, making small talk for a while. We were never sure if Grandma could remember how much time had passed between visits.

"Mom, I haven't been to visit for a few weeks, because Raymond has been very sick. Rae Ann has been helping me

take care of him." Mom paused for a moment, trying to hold back her tears. "*I am really sorry to tell you he died last week. Rae Ann has to go back to work, and she has asked me to stay with her for a few weeks so I don't have to be alone. I will miss you terribly, but you'll be well cared for here and I do want to stay with her. Will that be okay with you?*"

"Okay honey, don't be concerned about me," she smiled sweetly. "I'm fine here. Did you know they're going to have a piano concert today? I'm looking forward to it," she continued.

We sighed, not sure if she understood anything we told her, but certain she had forgotten the afternoon's entertainment was already over. About that time the staff started gathering people for the early dinner seating. Looking around, Grandma rose, smiling to give us each a hug. "It was so good to see you girls, but I need to go."

It wasn't fair to Mom, losing her husband and then having to say good-bye to her mother, but it was the best we could do. Caring for Mom was now my number-one priority.

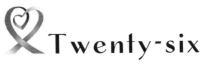

Twenty-six
Returning Home
November 29

Twenty-four days earlier I had arrived with one suitcase, packed with clothes for a week's visit. My stay was extended, I did my laundry frequently, and only once did I drive to the mall, run into JC Penney, and buy a pair of casual gray slacks and two long sleeve T-shirts to wear around the house. My new clothes fit easily into my suitcase and I was packed in less than twenty minutes. It was time to help Mom.

I carried Mom's large hardcover Samsonite suitcase in from the garage and placed it open on her bed, next to twenty large grapefruit she had carried in from the kitchen. Another reason Mom loved living in Palm Springs was being able to open her sliding glass door, take six steps and handpick fresh pink grapefruits from the tree that shaded their patio. I laughed as she placed each grapefruit in the suitcase. There wasn't much room left for clothes, but she didn't care. Dressing up and going out was not in her plans, but she did look forward to eating half a grapefruit every morning. I was delighted she was looking forward to anything.

Next she packed the photo album she put together earlier in the year, along with her small transistor radio, an eight-by-ten framed photo of Dad and her, her address book, and a small cloth bag filled with costume jewelry. She folded several pairs of panties, two bras, and four handkerchiefs, using them to pad the framed photo. She stood in front of her closet for a while, finally selecting two pairs of casual slacks, two long sleeve blouses, three short sleeve blouses, one sweatshirt, two nightgowns, a pair of slippers, and a cotton robe. On her bathroom counter she placed her Estee Lauder liquid make-up, mascara, eyeliner, eye shadow, eyebrow pencil, make-up remover, anti-wrinkle crème, Oil of Olay, Aim toothpaste, four toothbrushes, dental picks, floss, a comb, and her hairbrush. I packed them for her, reminding her I could buy anything she forgot or needed. Before shutting the suitcase she tossed in her meds.

I carried our suitcases, purses, and jackets to the entry hall while Mom moved from room to room, making sure the windows were shut, the blinds drawn, and the furnace set on fifty-five. She was wearing tennis shoes, navy slacks, a white blouse, white flower earrings, and her large dark sunglasses, this time perhaps more to hide her tears than for protection from the sun. Dad used to carry the suitcases, lock the front door, and help her into the car. Life had irrevocably changed, but there was no looking back as together we waited for our ride to the airport.

Twenty-seven
The Airport

Mom's girlfriend drove us to the Palm Springs International Airport, another sad good-bye. The good news was we were dropped off right in front of the Alaska Airlines ticket counter. We walked through the glass sliding doors and I escorted Mom to an empty row of seats, where she people-watched while I checked in our two bags and obtained our boarding passes.

I encouraged Mom to use a wheelchair to avoid the long walk to the boarding gate, but she said no. Sometimes pride is a good thing; other times it gets in the way of giving the body needed rest.

We eventually made our way through security and down the lengthy corridor to the gate, boarded the airplane, found our seats, and stowed our purses for our one-hour flight to San Francisco. It had been more than twenty years since Mom and I had been on a plane together. Under different circumstances, we would have been talking and having fun, but instead we were quiet. I imagined Mom thinking how strange it was to be traveling without her husband, or how strange it felt to not have a husband any longer; but she didn't complain.

Mom took the window seat while I settled into the aisle seat. The sky was clear, allowing her to reminisce about driving trips with Dad along the roads below, as she looked down over the stunning

Carmel and Monterey coastline. Our dinner was a glass of tomato juice and a bag of peanuts.

We landed and taxied to our gate at the San Francisco International Airport. By the time we gathered our purses and jackets, made our way off the airplane and started walking to the baggage claim area, I could tell that Mom was physically tired.

"Mom," I said, leaning her way, "would you like a wheelchair?"

"*No,*" she grimaced, as if to say, "I can do it."

I should have insisted on a wheelchair, because by the time we slowly walked past four other gates, the security entrance, rode down two sets of escalators, turned right and walked past three baggage carousels, she was exhausted. I saw an empty row of chairs against the wall and helped her into one. I put our purses in the seat next to her and pulled out a zip-lock bag filled with ice and one Ensure.

A few weeks earlier, in my quest to bring humor to a sad time, I bought Mom a plastic sixteen-ounce drinking glass decorated with Mickey and Minnie Mouse, wearing bright red and green clothing, with distinctive yellow shoes. Mom was now drinking one Ensure daily, both for calories and energy, and to make her daily drink fun, I would pour it into this cute children's cup. It was lightweight, with a bright blue lid and straw. I bought it during one of my trips to the grocery store, with the hope that it would make

Mom laugh, which it did. It also turned out to be practical.

I pulled the cup out of my purse and poured the chocolate Ensure into it. Tightening the lid, I handed it to Mom. I tossed the empty zip-lock bag into a nearby trashcan on my way to the baggage carousel, ready to claim our luggage as it came down the chute.

I glanced over to check on Mom when I didn't think she was looking my way. She looked tired and a little frightened, sitting alone, drinking Ensure out of that silly cup. I was becoming the parent and we both knew it.

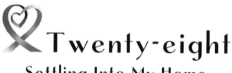

Twenty-eight
Settling Into My Home

Mill Valley was home to John Muir, the naturalist and founder of the Sierra Club. The center of the town is built around what was once a functioning railroad station. I used to enjoy going to the Depot, a popular place to eat breakfast or lunch, buy books, and watch people.

Mom and I made the one-hour ride home via the Marin Airporter shuttle, which offers scheduled service between the airport and various drop-off points in Marin County. Their easily identifiable white buses, with large colorful rainbows painted on the sides, are roomy with comfortable reclining seats and large windows. The bus stopped close to my condo, where a cab was waiting and drove us the short ride home.

I bought my townhouse because it was a short three-mile drive to my office and I liked the fact that my bedroom and the living room overlooked a narrow arm of the San Francisco bay. The condos, designed to look like Cape Cod homes, were unique to the area. Weaving through our cluster of townhouses was a paved walking path for the public to enjoy. Throughout the days and evenings, locals would drive to Shelter Bay, park their cars, then briskly walk or stroll down the path. Many were with dogs, seeking exercise; some were bird watching; and the rest enjoyed other outdoor pleasures.

My townhouse was about 1,500 square feet, with two bedrooms, two bathrooms and the washer and dryer upstairs. The galley kitchen, half bath, dining room, and living room were on the main level. The oak wood floors in the entry hall, dining room, and kitchen, the wood trim on the short wall dividing the dining room from the step-down living room, and the off-white carpet throughout the rest of the house caught my eye when the realtor first showed me the unit. After it became my home, I would enter through the connected two-car garage, but guests made their way to the front door by walking through a small, treed courtyard shared by three other units.

The stairs leading up to the bedrooms were opposite the dining room, left of the front entry and guest bath. My bedroom, at the top of the stairs and directly above the living room, was a good size room, big enough for my queen bed, one nightstand, and a desk for my computer and files. The large bathroom inside my bedroom contained mirrored closets, a bathtub, and a shower. Even before Mom came to live with me, I spent most of my time in my bedroom, either working or resting. It was a cozy room, with one large window to view the bay and the public walkway.

Walking out of my bedroom, I could make a slight turn right and go back down the stairs, or walk straight down the hall, no more than twenty steps, to the guest room. Between the bedrooms on the left, hidden behind pull-out louvered doors, were shelves I used to store my sheets, blankets, and towels, next to the full-size washer and dryer. Just before entering the guest room, on the right, was a bathroom with a large walk-in shower.

Mom and I arrived Sunday night, about eight. After unlocking the front door, turning on the lights, and making sure Mom was safely in the house, I was thrilled to see my kittens run to the front door to greet us. They seemed to have grown during the month I was away, and even better, they acted like they remembered me, which made me happy.

We looked around, pleasantly surprised to find vases filled with colorful flowers throughout the house. There was a small bouquet on the kitchen table, one on the dining room table, and a larger arrangement in my bathroom upstairs. Along with the flowers was a card, signed by each person in my office, welcoming us home and reminding us that they were there to support us. The flowers and card were exactly what we needed, a reminder that we were not alone.

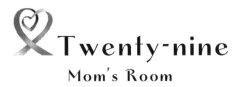

Twenty-nine
Mom's Room

Mom settled into the guest room. Her bedroom was smaller than mine, but large enough for a queen-size bed, a wicker headboard, and two matching wicker nightstands. The bed was centered between windows that I opened in the summer to bring in the salt-water breeze. Against the wall opposite the foot of the bed, nestled between the open door and the walk-in closet, was a seven-foot tall maple bookcase, its four shelves filled with knickknacks, books, and a thirteen-inch screen TV. In the summer, looking out through the large picture window I could see a tall purple leaf plum tree that shaded a good portion of the bedroom. Earlier in the year that tree was the first in the area to bloom, covered in pale pink flowers. By the time Mom moved in, the tree was dormant, its deep reddish leaves having fallen the prior month. I was hopeful she would live to see it bloom the next spring.

I had neither the time nor the money to change the off-white aluminum mini blinds or paint the interior walls; living with the Swiss Coffee color selected by the previous owners was fine with me. Soon after moving in I had purchased an eight-piece queen comforter set on sale. The reversible yellow comforter with the pink, blue and green flowers, and matching bed skirt and pillow shams brightened the guest room. At local festivals I had purchased colorful posters, which after framing were hung on the walls. The blue framed Mill Valley poster was on the wall to the left of the doorway, the red frame celebrating Sausalito was hanging on the far right wall, just left of the picture window, and the yellow framed poster of the vineyards of Napa was centered above the bed.

I placed Mom's suitcase on the yellow flowered bedspread and opened it so she could unpack. First she carefully removed the framed color photo of Dad and her, smiling because the glass was not broken, and placed it on the bookcase for her viewing pleasure. The picture had been taken at one of Dad's high school reunions. My guess is they were probably about sixty in the picture. I don't know if it was Mom's favorite picture because they had enjoyed a fun evening that night, or because she liked the red outfit she was wearing, or because her hair looked good, or because she thought Dad looked particularly handsome in the photo. I never asked her because the reason didn't matter; we all knew it was her favorite picture.

Her next concern was unpacking the grapefruit and getting them into the refrigerator. I made several trips up and down the stairs, kittens at my feet, before all twenty grapefruit were in the kitchen. Opening the refrigerator, I was thrilled to see that my neighbor, Anitah, had bought us a jug of one-percent milk, wheat bread, half and half for my morning coffee, and orange juice. My refrigerator bins each held five grapefruit. I stacked the other ten on the shelves, nearly filling the inside.

Mom placed her treasured photo album she had made, filled with her favorite pictures taken during fifty-two years of marriage, on the nightstand, next to her transistor radio and the digital clock, with its large green numbers easy to read in the middle of the night. In the bathroom she opened the medicine cabinet, lined up her cosmetics, made sure that the labels faced outward, and borrowed my extra glass container of cotton balls that she placed under the sink. She stored her jewelry in the bottom drawer, tooth products in the middle drawer, and hairbrush and comb in the top drawer.

After taking out her slippers and nightgown, she asked me to close the suitcase and store it under her bed. I understood her wanting to avoid the closet where she used to hang the clothes she and Dad planned to wear during their visits. She changed into her nightgown, took her sleeping pill, removed her make-up, brushed and flossed her teeth, finally crawling into bed. I walked into her room, to make sure she was comfortable in her new surroundings. We kissed, and I turned off the light, leaving her bedroom door open in case she needed me later in the evening. I was grateful to have spent one more day with Mom, not knowing how many more days we would share.

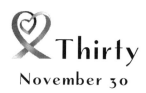

Thirty

November 30

I planned to leave early for the office Monday morning. Mom heard me getting ready and got up to say good-bye. After refreshing in the bathroom, she snuggled back into bed, turning on her nightstand lamp, enjoying my waiting on her. I brought her the *San Francisco Chronicle* and a cup of hot black coffee, placing them both on the nightstand beside her address book, telephone, and box of Kleenex for that persistent cough.

"If you feel up to it later today," I suggested, "maybe you can call some of your friends to tell them we arrived safely." Mom loved to connect with friends, via telephone or mail. Neither she nor Dad had a computer, and even though I explained how easy it was to communicate via email, she had no desire to learn.

"*Don't worry about me,*" she smiled. "*After you leave I'll read for awhile, and later go downstairs to fix my breakfast, then make some calls.*"

She didn't have much of an appetite, but at least I knew she would eat half a grapefruit.

"Super. I'll call you when I can break for lunch," I said. "I plan to stop at the grocery store, then come home and fix us a bite."

With my hair twisted up and held with a black claw clip, make-up applied, wearing a white blouse, short black jacket with matching skirt and high heels,I was dressed for the office. Before leaving, I leaned over to give Mom a morning "I love you" hug. The kittens had already jumped on her bed and were playing with each other, making Mom laugh.

I didn't like leaving her, but I needed to be back in the office. My continuing thought was to do what I needed to keep my promise to Mom. I still wanted to be just like her, so I did my best to live for each day and not think too far ahead.

Work was a good release for me. At the office I could be in control, negotiate a better deal, analyze a problem, discuss it with others, and together we could solve it. I had great team support. I could make decisions and make things happen.

At home it was the exact opposite. I couldn't make things better. I couldn't stop Dad from leaving us and I couldn't stop Mom's cancer from spreading. Outside of the office I had no support, no brothers or sisters, no family in the area. The only decisions I could make were related to what we would eat, and even then Mom often refused my selections.

It was good to be back at work. One by one, people came into my office to give me hugs and offers of support. I was blessed to have an understanding boss and colleagues. But, business is business and soon I felt like I had never left. Between conference calls, meetings, contracts to review, and weeks of mail to read, the time passed quickly.

I wasn't able to get out of the office until one that afternoon. I stopped at Mollie Stone's grocery store deli on my way home and picked up a turkey sandwich to share with Mom. I was back in the office by two and ended up working until after seven. Too tired to cook dinner, for the second time that day I stopped at Mollie Stone's, this time bringing home chicken vegetable soup and fresh sourdough rolls. By the time we finished eating it was nearly nine. We were both in bed early that night, glad to leave the month of November behind.

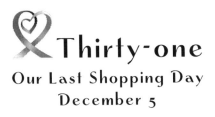

Thirty-one

Our Last Shopping Day
December 5

I was noticing a new pattern. One day Mom would feel okay, but the next day she would not be well and would rest much more. Then she might feel well for two days in a row, followed by a third day of exhaustion.

Fortunately, Saturday morning she was feeling fine and asked if we could go shopping at the local mall, just a few miles north. I quickly answered, "Yes!" The two anchor stores were Macy's on the south and Nordstrom on the north end, with plenty of specialty shops in between. I was thrilled Mom wanted to go out.

It was after eleven before we were ready to leave. The sun was shining when I backed the car out of the garage. As the garage door closed, Mom took her large sunglasses out of her purse, slipped them on, and flipped down the visor to check her appearance. We got on the freeway, then off at the first exit, surprised to find the parking lots already full. I stopped in the loading zone in front of Nordstrom, got out, and walked around to the passenger door to help Mom out of the car.

"Mom, why don't you sit on this bench while I drive around and try to find a parking space? I might have to park far away, and instead of you walking back with me, I'd prefer you wait here." (I was glad she was wearing one of my warm coats.) Mom nodded in agreement.

"I can't believe I didn't realize the mall would be packed with holiday shoppers," I said. "After all, it is the first weekend in December, but since we agreed we're not going to celebrate Christmas, I guess I put the holiday season out of my thoughts."

"I don't mind waiting for you, you know how I love to people watch. And since we aren't going to celebrate this year, it's nice to see the colorful decorations."

I ended up having to park on an overflow gravel parking lot, a long walk from where I left her. She waved as I approached.

"Honey, I don't know how long I'll feel like shopping. Do you mind if we start in Nordstrom?"

"That works for me," I replied. "Let's look around, eat lunch, and then see how you feel."

We worked our way through the crowds in Nordstrom, moving through the shoe department on our way around the first floor. I left her for a short time, wanting to look at business suits on the second floor. On my way down the escalator I spotted Mom in the jewelry department, leaning on a glass cabinet looking at necklaces and rings. My once tall, strong, and vibrant mother appeared stooped, weary and frail. The physical decline I had noticed the prior week at the airport was even more pronounced. November had taken the wind out of her sails.

I wanted to bring joy back into her life, but I couldn't bring back Dad or make her healthy again. I wanted to scream and cry as the reality that I would soon lose her too was almost unbearable. But it was my turn to be the strong one and take care of her, so I replaced my heartache with a smile, walked up behind her, slipped my arms around her thinning waist, and whispered, "I love you so much. Thanks for staying with me."

Good to go one more day.

As I had expected, Mom rested most of Sunday and Monday. Our shopping excursion had taken its toll, however, she didn't feel very well on Tuesday either; nor did she want to eat much more than her half grapefruit and one Ensure. I was constantly nagging her to eat.

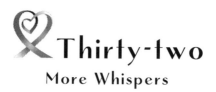

Thirty-two
More Whispers

The whispers were back, urging me to call hospice for Mom. This time there would be no opposition. Both of us were amazed by the care they provided for Dad and the support and care they gave to Mom and me during that twenty-four hour period.

At home, I dug through the many papers on my desk and found the notes of my October 18th phone call with Vickie. It was hard to believe we had talked less than six weeks ago; it seemed an eternity.

In reading my notes, one line was prominent: "Connect with hospice as soon as possible." Those were the words of my whispers. I wondered how I would know when it was the right time to call.

On Wednesday, during my lunch break, I called to check in on Mom. Her voice was weak and she didn't feel well. She hadn't eaten, the radio and TV were off, and she planned to sleep the rest of the day. I hung up, upset and sad, walked over to shut my office door, took a deep breath and called Hospice of Marin.

The lady who answered asked me several questions. Once again I told our story. She wanted our address and the name of Mom's doctor. After learning that Mom's doctor was in Palm Desert, she explained that a doctor in Marin County had to see Mom in order to confirm that she was ready for hospice.Darn, now I would have to locate a doctor who would accept a new patient, make an appointment, take more time off work, pick Mom up, drive her to the doctor's office and drive her back home.

I sighed and asked if she could recommend a local doctor and was surprised when she said she would send one directly to our home. What a relief. The doctor would be out the following week, but they could send a hospice nurse to see Mom that afternoon or the following morning. I wanted to be sure Mom was in agreement, so we scheduled an appointment for eleven the following morning.

That night after work Mom and I talked about hospice coming to see her. She agreed it would be a good idea to talk with them and get their thoughts on her lack of energy and care. We agreed it would be good for me too, because I might receive guidance on how to make her more comfortable. At least one good thing had come from Dad's passing, we knew who to call for exceptionally good help.

Photographs and Memories

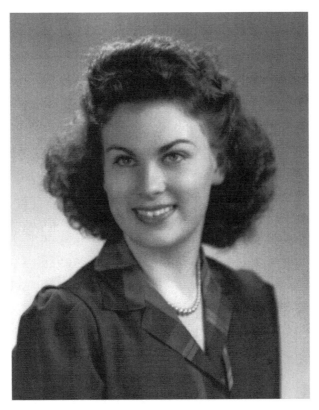

Mom, Anne Berry, at age 19

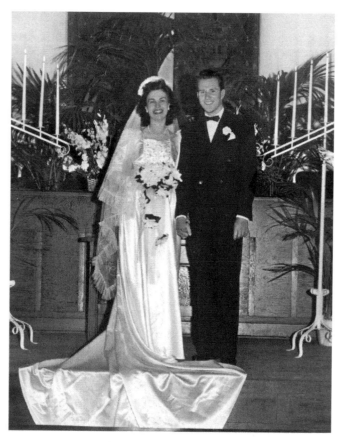

Mom and Dad on their wedding day
June 1, 1946

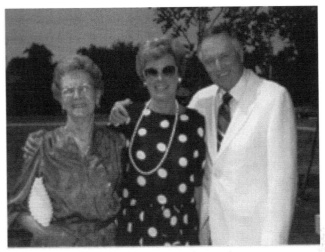

Grandma, Mom, and Dad - 1982

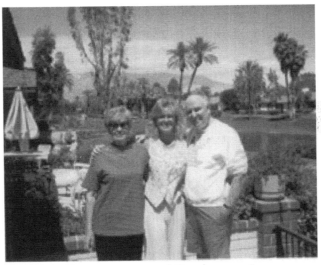

Mom, me, and Dad - 1996

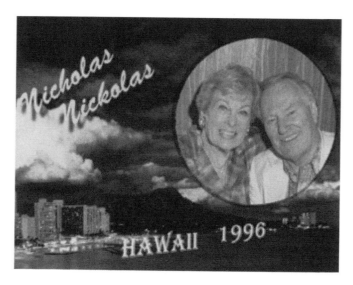

50th wedding anniversary

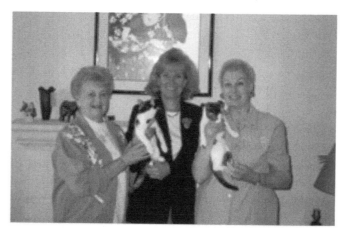

Adele, me, Mom, and the kittens - 1998

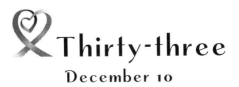

Thirty-three

December 10

Thursday morning, I worked from home. I hadn't slept well, having mixed emotions about calling hospice again. On one hand, I wasn't ready to acknowledge that Mom might be leaving soon, but it was clear she was getting worse. On the other hand, I was scared hospice might say she wasn't ready for their care, and then where would I turn for guidance and support.

That morning, after coffee and her half grapefruit, Mom washed her face, brushed her teeth, carefully applied her make-up, put on earrings and lipstick, then dressed in a casual top and slacks before getting back into bed. I was downstairs in the kitchen when I heard a car out front. I ran to the garden window, leaned over, and turned my head to the right to get a close look at the driver. I saw a tall lady step out of a dark station wagon. Her long slightly graying brunette hair was braided, ending in a ponytail that ran midway down her back. She was wearing a gray top with black slacks, black clogs, and carried a medical bag.

I ran up the stairs and yelled, "She's here!" then ran back down the stairs to greet the nurse. When I opened the front door I was struck by that same soft, calm feeling that Dorothy had given me. The lady at the door looked a little older than me, perhaps in her early fifties.

"Hello, you must be Rae Ann. My name is Peggy. I'm a nurse with Hospice of Marin. May I come in?"

"Please do," I smiled, holding out my hand to shake hers. "Thank you for coming to see us."

"It's our pleasure," she replied. "We're glad you called. I understand you've already used hospice services for your father."

I nodded in reply.

"I'm so very sorry for your loss," she said. "Do you want to talk with me, or would you like to join me while I speak with your Mother?"

"I'd love to listen while you talk to Mom," I replied. "That is, if you don't mind."

Peggy smiled. By now the kittens had run down the stairs, one sniffing the bottom of her slacks, and the other smelling her medical bag.

"I hope you aren't allergic to cats," I laughed.

"No," she replied. "I'm always happy to see pets in a home. They're very instinctive, and they seem to know when to comfort those who aren't well. And, at a time like this," she added, "their love goes a long way."

Peggy followed me up the stairs and into Mom's room. I thought Mom looked pretty sitting in her bed, with her make-up and lipstick freshly applied. I wasn't sure whether Peggy would realize just how ill she was. Although she was often tired and struggled with that ever-present cough, Mom could still eat, walk, talk, shower and use the bathroom on her own.

Oh yes, there was that new growth on the right side of her face, halfway between her forehead and her eyebrow. It didn't stick out more than a half-inch—about the size of my little fingernail—and although it had appeared quickly, Mom said it didn't hurt, which was our primary concern. It reminded me of a unicorn's horn, which is what we called it to make us laugh. Mom thought that her growth was located in the perfect spot, since it didn't bother her day or night, even though she liked to sleep on her stomach. Funny thing; those body cells gone haywire. They really did spell cancer wrong—four letters would have been sufficient.

After introductions, Mom smiled and welcomed Peggy into her room. I stood in the doorway as Peggy sat down and placed her medical bag on her lap, faced Mom and asked how she was feeling. Peggy was a good listener, letting Mom talk about her life, her health, and Dad.

Once it was clear that Mom felt comfortable, Peggy asked if she minded my leaving them alone so that she could examine her.

"*Yes, that's fine,*" Mom replied, nodding her head as if granting me permission to leave the room. Before I turned around to leave, Peggy had stood, placed her medical bag on the chair, taken the stethoscope out of her medical bag, placed the ear tips in her ears, twisted them to make a seal, and was gently placing the chestpiece against Mom's lungs.

Thirty minutes later I heard Mom calling me. I passed Peggy in Mom's bathroom, washing her hands.

Before leaving, Peggy handed me a pamphlet, suggesting that later we take time to read through the information that would help us understand what to expect as Mom's body slowly shut down. She turned to Mom.

"It's a pleasure to get to know you Anne. If you have any questions, please call me. Assuming Dr. Hand finds you are appropriate for our hospice program, I'd like to visit again next week. Would that be okay with you?"

"*Of course,*" replied Mom. "*Anytime you want to visit is fine with me. I'll be here. Thank you again for coming.*"

As I walked Peggy to her car, she shared some of their conversation with me. Mom had told her that she hoped she could die quickly because I had already been through so much sadness the past month, and with my working long hours and a stressful job, I didn't need to also be worrying about her.

"She said she doesn't want to be a burden," Peggy said, "and that she really doesn't want to be in a hospital or a nursing home. She's praying to leave quickly."

Peggy had assured Mom that I was grateful she was with me, and that she and the other hospice workers would be there to support me.

I wanted Peggy's medical opinion about Mom's health, so I asked. "Based on examining and talking with Mom, how long do you think she has left to live?"

"We don't like to give a time estimate," she replied, "because so many times we're incorrect. Sometimes, after people start receiving hospice care, they feel so much better that they live quite a while longer." I nodded with hope.

"Through the years we've learned that everyone's body is different. The way a disease affects one person may be entirely different than the way it affects another person. Please understand, your mother could live much longer than five or six weeks or she could die sooner. We just can't tell. I'm telling you my best guess, based on what I observed and how she told me she feels."

I walked back to the house taking a few deep breaths, still shaking inside after hearing Peggy's confirmation that Mom's body was failing her, just as I had suspected. The kittens ran down the stairs to greet me. I bent over to pet them both, and then ran up the stairs, with the cats following closely behind, to hear her thoughts about Peggy.

I remembered Vickie telling me that if we didn't get along with our hospice nurse or anyone else sent over by hospice, we could call and ask for someone else. Vickie said they understood that sometimes personalities just don't mix. I was very comfortable with Peggy, and I hoped Mom felt the same way.

"Well Mom, what did you think about Peggy?"

"Oh honey; what a nice lady. She has that soft, uplifting, lyrical voice that Dorothy had, don't you think? She listened to me and seems to think I am doing fine. Did you hear her say she wants to see me again next week after the new doctor checks me out? Oh, and would you mind

getting me some V8 juice now? I'm a little thirsty. Then I think I'll read a little and then have a rest, because I don't want to miss Judge Judy at four. Thanks honey. I'm so sorry to be such a burden to you."

"Mom, you're not a burden," I told her. "I love you with all my heart. I'd rather have you in my home, where we can talk, and laugh, and share time together, and where I know you're comfortable and well cared for. Working as much as I am, it'd be hard for me to have to drive to an assisted living home or hospital every time I wanted to see you. I'd hate waking up in the night and not being able to walk down the hall to check on you. I love knowing you're in my house. You cared for me; now let me care for you."

Thirty-four
The Doctor Visit
December 15

Hospice called me at the office the following Tuesday to tell me that Dr. Hand, an oncologist in the area, would be coming to see Mom later that afternoon. I still couldn't believe that the doctor was going to come to our house. How wonderful was that? I made sure I was home early to meet him.

I didn't expect we would see Dr. Hand again after this visit, so I wasn't concerned about his looks or whether or not we connected with him. When I opened the front door I was surprised to see a very attractive, well-dressed lady standing before me.

Shame on me for presuming Dr. Hand was a man.

I walked her upstairs to meet Mom, who was sitting up in bed, wearing make up, lipstick, and earrings, looking forward to meeting someone new. After introducing Dr. Hand, I left Mom's room so the doctor could talk with her and examine her. She had already reviewed Mom's medical history.

Dr. Hand agreed Mom was appropriate for hospice and told us that Peggy would visit the next day. Mom and I were both relieved that hospice had agreed to help us, although neither one of us stated the obvious—that Mom wouldn't be returning to the desert.

I walked Dr. Hand downstairs.

"I'm so sorry to hear of your dad's recent passing," she said quietly. "Dealing with his loss, working full time, and now caring for your mom is going to be very difficult. Please find quiet time to take care of yourself and remember that hospice provides many services, including someone for you to talk through your concerns and feelings. I know this is new for you, but we have years of experience, so please don't be shy about reaching out for assistance."

I have learned that being a caregiver is extremely hard work; it is physically, mentally, and emotionally draining. In hindsight I should have listened to her, and on certain days, I should have taken better care of myself. I have learned that a tired caregiver is of little value to the patient.

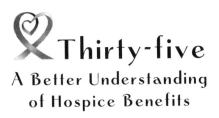

Thirty-five
A Better Understanding of Hospice Benefits

The next day, Peggy came back to the house to enroll Mom in the hospice program, this time accompanied by Joe, a tall, slender man about my age wearing khaki Dockers, deck shoes, and a long-sleeved light blue shirt. He was a counselor, and his job was to be there for Mom and me, to listen, and to answer our non-medical questions. If we needed to vent, we could call him. What a benefit to have our own counselor, at no expense.

Peggy and Joe politely explained that they would like to spend time with Mom, then visited with her for about thirty minutes before calling me to join them. Peggy needed some further information, so I showed her Mom's Medicare and supplemental insurance cards. In addition, she and Dad were members of the Neptune Society, having decided years earlier that they wanted to be cremated, and I provided that information as well. After making her notes, Peggy handed Mom the clipboard so she could sign the required forms for admission to the Hospice of Marin program.

Holding the signed paperwork in her lap, Peggy turned her attention to me where I sat next to Mom.

"Your mom told us that she doesn't have an appetite, and we want you to know it's okay if she doesn't want to eat. As the physical body shuts down, it doesn't need as much food as it once required. Because your mom is resting in bed all day, her body needs even less to sustain it. It's natural for you to want to see your mom eat, but please know it's okay if she just wants something sweet or a piece of toast. Whether or not she wants to eat is her decision, and we should honor that decision."

I felt a bit admonished but nodded with consent, guessing that Mom had told them I was constantly nagging her to eat.

"We also talked with your mom about a few other things," Peggy said, "and she's made some other decisions."

I took a silent breath.

"She'd like us to order medication to relieve her depression and to calm her when she becomes anxious," she said. "Understandably, the recent death of your father, combined with her declining health, has caused her to be down, and it's common that patients with breathing difficulties become anxious."

I nodded again, taking in all of this new information.

Peggy further explained that one of the side effects of the medications was constipation, but she said she could order another pill to take care of it and offered to call in each prescription before she and Joe left. I was relieved to find out that they would be delivered to my door in only a few hours; I was also happy when Peggy said she'd order a raised seat for the toilet, to make it easier for Mom to push herself up. "It'll be delivered later today," she said, "along with a walker and a shower chair. We can also send a home health aide to bathe your mom if she likes."

Though I felt comforted by all of the care, Peggy must have sensed my concern that these extra essentials were suddenly necessary.

"Your mom told us that she doesn't have the energy to walk up and down the stairs," she said with compassion. "She says she's a bit wobbly on her feet, and the walker will make her steady. She's also too weak to stand in the shower. That's why we're going to order a shower chair, so she can continue to shower on her own. And if it's okay with you, I'd like to come back to see her early next week."

I had to admit that her words surprised me. I was not aware that Mom was depressed, anxious, or struggling to walk, but I tried not to show it. I was grateful for their expertise and assistance; I would have never known which medications and equipment would help Mom.

"Of course we want you back anytime," I said with a smile, "but before you go, could I ask a favor?"

"Sure," Peggy said.

"If you have a little extra time, do you think you could tell Mom and me more about hospice? We didn't really have time to learn with Dad." I glanced at Mom. "I guess we were in crisis mode."

Peggy nodded, knowing exactly what I meant. "We'd be happy to."

Mom and I listened intently as Peggy explained that hospice is a type of care for people who have life-limiting illnesses, such as cancer, advanced lung disease, heart disease, kidney disease, or any illness that is estimated to reduce a life span to a period of six months or less. We learned that though it is not uncommon for a person to go on hospice care and live a year or longer, other people actually improve to the point where they're released from the program for a period of time.

"Our experience has shown that the sooner a person receives hospice care," Joe said, "the better their quality of life becomes."

"But whether to accept hospice care is an individual decision," Joe continued. "When faced with a life-threatening illness, some people would prefer to fight with all their might. They seek aggressive treatment, while others don't want any treatment and prefer to continue with life until the disease slowly ends their quality of life. Many people take the path in the middle, initially choosing treatment of some form."

I glanced at Mom and saw that she was looking down in thought. I wondered if she was thinking about Dad.

I looked at Peggy. "What if someone wants to choose aggressive treatment, like chemo? Are they ineligible for hospice?"

"Not at this point," Peggy said. "But we expect that might change in the future. The thing is, hospice really focuses on the care, not the cure, of the patient and their caregivers. Our goal is to make each patient comfortable and free from pain so they're able to live each day to the fullest."

I nodded and smiled, admiring their mission. "So how did it get started?"

Peggy explained that the name actually originated long ago when a "hospice" was shelter for travelers where they could find care, comfort, and support during their journey. In 1967, Dame Cicely Saunders, an English doctor and well-known leader in the hospice movement, opened St. Christopher's Hospice in a London suburb, focusing on pain and symptom relief, to meet the physical, social, psychological, and spiritual needs of patients and their families and friends. Dame Saunders is quoted as saying: "You matter because you are you and you matter to the last moment of your life. We will do all we can not only to help you die peacefully, but to live until you die." That care became the model for hospices around the world.

"The first hospice in the United States was founded in 1974 in Branford, Connecticut," Peggy said. "Our hospice, Hospice of Marin, is the second oldest one in the United States, founded in 1975. In 1982, the United States Congress made hospice a Medicare covered benefit. Last year, in 1997, there were approximately 3,000 hospice programs nationwide, and it's now estimated that hospices will care for about 540,000, or one quarter of the people who'll die this year."

I looked at Peggy wide-eyed, stunned by the statistics. "So is it mainly for the elderly, then, who have Medicare?"

"Actually, no," she said. "Anyone, young or old, is eligible. If the patient qualifies for Medicare, then the service is paid for by Medicare. But many insurance plans now cover it too."

"That's wonderful," I said. Mom nodded in agreement.

"The thing we want to remind people," Peggy said, "is that hospice care neither prolongs nor hastens life."

Mom and I looked at each other and smiled.

Joe then added that hospice services included more than we probably realized: nursing care, medical equipment, medical supplies, medication, home health aide care, social worker services, patient and family counseling throughout the patient's care, and a year of bereavement counseling for the family after the patient's death. "In most jurisdictions," he said, "hospice services are provided wherever the patient resides, whether at their home, in a nursing home, or in a hospital, and many areas also have hospice facilities."

"But how do people learn about hospice?" I asked. "We only heard of it through a friend of a friend."

Joe nodded. "Well, generally the patient's doctor and sometimes the hospital will tell the patient and the family about hospice. Since doctors are trained to cure people, some may feel as if they've failed if they acknowledge a patient has a short period of time left to live. But," he added with enthusiasm, "doctors are now seeing the many benefits that hospice provides the patient and the family, and they're learning that giving information about hospice gives the patient the opportunity to make a reasoned decision about whether to continue treatment or to turn to hospice for palliative care."

"My daughter refers to hospice as 'comfort care,'" Mom said. *"I used to love cooking her favorite meal of roast chicken and mashed potatoes, which she calls 'comfort food.' Now she thinks of hospice and the comfort it provided us when my husband was dying. So would referring to palliative care as 'comfort care' be accurate?"*

Both Peggy and Joe smiled. "Yes, Anne. Perfectly."

Mom smiled in return.

Not wanting to take too much of their time, I took my cue to end our conversation on that positive note. I patted Mom on the leg. "Well, this has been really enlightening," I said. "Mom thinks I ask too many questions, so I'll stop for now." I shot Mom a playful glance, then turned back to Peggy and Joe. "Thank you so much for taking the time to share all this information with us."

"Our pleasure," Peggy said with a warm smile, gathering her things. "I'll be back next week, but in the meantime, if you need to see me or talk to me, just call and leave me a message. I check my messages throughout the day, and I'll find time to be available anytime you need me."

"Thank you so much," I said.

"And in case Peggy isn't available right away," Joe added, "you can call and talk to a hospice nurse any time, day or night, if you have questions."

"That's great," I said, noticing Mom was smiling.

Peggy and Joe told me they were fine to show themselves out while I stayed to talk with Mom, so we said our good-byes upstairs. After they were gone, I apologized to Mom for trying to make her eat when she wasn't hungry.

"It's okay," she said. *"I know you're just trying to take care of me."*

While Mom rested, I worked from home. Just before four, I heard Mom's TV and smiled. At least I could still count on two things: every day she would eat a half grapefruit; and each weekday she would watch *Judge Judy,* one of the first reality TV shows, featuring a former family court judge who arbitrated small claims court cases.

The doorbell rang twice that afternoon. The first time it was a deliveryman, who handed me the raised toilet seat, the shower chair, and the walker. I didn't even have to sign a receipt. Mom was skeptical about the raised toilet seat, but I set it in place and tried it first. After it had my seal of approval, she agreed to use it.

The second visitor was a young delivery boy from the local pharmacy. He handed me a white bag, filled with three prescriptions. I asked him what I owed. "Nothing, it's paid for," he said. I found that amazing.

I had also called a handyman who was able to come over later that evening. I explained that Mom needed a shower chair and asked if he could change the permanent shower head to one she could hold in her hand while she rinsed. He knew exactly what I wanted. When he arrived, he also brought a chrome bar that he installed on the side of the shower so that

Mom had something to hold onto while getting in and out. It was much easier for her to enjoy the shower if she wasn't tired from standing or afraid of falling.

While all of these additions were helpful, I admit we accepted some changes that were best for Mom more readily than others.

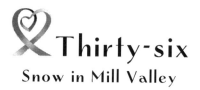

Thirty-six
Snow in Mill Valley

After staying in bed a few days Mom was looking forward to a long, warm shower. I helped her out of bed, placed the walker in front of her, and with my assistance, we shuffled the fifteen feet from her bed to her bathroom. I helped her to undress and sit safely on the shower chair, and then handed her the nozzle and turned on the water, which I had warmed a few minutes earlier. She was able to hold onto the bar with her right hand and shower with her left hand.

I stood in the hall outside her bathroom, playing with the kittens, ready to help her if she needed me. I could hear her moaning with delight as she ran the heated water over her body. I glanced outside and saw that it was raining. After a few minutes at my post, having thrown several little red balls down the hall for the kittens, I looked outside again. I could not believe my eyes. It was snowing!

I wanted to share the experience with Mom, who was from Southern California, where snow is quite rare. I was so excited that I didn't think; instead, I yelled at her to come out and see the snow. She cut her shower short, grabbed her towel, and with my help wobbled to the hall and looked outside. She saw about ten seconds of snow falling, and then it turned back to rain. We were both amazed to see the snowflakes, but had I known by drawing attention to the snow I was cutting short what would be Mom's last shower, I would have watched the snow in silence.

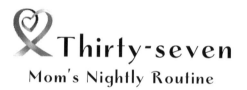

Thirty-seven
Mom's Nightly Routine

For more than fifty years, before Mom went to sleep, her routine had been to remove her make-up, wash her face, apply her face cream, brush her teeth, floss, and brush her hair. By the third week of December she was too weak to walk into the bathroom and stand for this process; so each night I helped her do all of these things while she was in bed.

I placed her make-up remover, cotton balls, Oil of Olay, toothpaste, toothbrush, floss, hairbrush, a washcloth, and a towel on a tray, and then carried the tray to her room. Next, I would hold Mom's outstretched hands and gently pull her forward into a sitting position (which took patience on my part and energy on hers), placing five pillows behind her back. Moving her into a sitting position caused a lot of coughing, so we always kept Kleenex and a wastebasket next to the bed.

Once she was sitting up, I would hand her the cotton balls and make-up remover. While she was taking off her make-up, I would go downstairs, fill a pot with warm water, and bring it to her. She'd rinse the washcloth, scrub her face, and repeat the process several times. Next I would hand Mom a towel to dry her face, and then hand her the Oil of Olay to apply while I went to the bathroom to throw out the warm water and rinse the washcloth, which I then tossed in the laundry basket. I would carry the pot downstairs, wash it, dry it, and fill it with cold water before I brought it back. I'd take her toothbrush, apply toothpaste, dip the toothbrush in the water, and then give it to Mom, holding the pot over her lap while she brushed her teeth. When she was finished, I would give her a glass of water to drink and then hand her the floss. While she flossed, I would take the toothpaste, toothbrush, make-up remover, and Oil of Olay back into the bathroom and put them away.

By then she would have finished brushing her hair. I'd hand her whatever pills she needed with a glass of water, making sure to record in the notebook the day, the time, and the medications I handed her. She'd sit up a bit more, so that I would then remove the five pillows and place my hands on her shoulder to support her while she slowly lay back into her sleeping position. Leaning over the side of her bed, I'd give her a kiss and whisper, "I love you," as I turned off the bedroom light.

At the end of the hall, I'd pick up the pot and carry it downstairs, wondering how long we would continue to share our nightly routine. While washing, rinsing and drying the pot, I would became lost in thought, thinking of all I had to do before I could crawl into bed. I had to tend to the kittens, then, it was my turn to take off my make-up, brush my teeth, floss, and dress for bed.

Turning away from the kitchen sink, I would see it behind me--that irritating form. One of the hospice forms Mom had signed was a DNR, "Do Not Resuscitate." We had many discussions and were in total agreement that our goal was for Mom to die comfortably at home. She did not want to be resuscitated nor moved to a hospital. A difficult situation could arise if I were away from the house, while someone else was watching Mom. They might call 911, resulting in the paramedics coming to the house. In Marin County, paramedics would not resuscitate someone without first checking the refrigerator door, where an active DNR was to be placed.

Each night, as I saw that DNR form, two Golden Gate Bridge magnets holding it on my refrigerator door, I heard it shouting, "Your best friend, your mom, is dying!" (As if I didn't know.)

I was starting to hate that form. I had plans for it.

Thirty-eight

Energy Units

The days passed slowly. Mom had less and less energy and went from sleeping eight hours a day to sleeping twelve to fourteen hours a day. I called hospice and asked Peggy to come over; maybe she would have suggestions on how I should better care for Mom.

Peggy explained that when a body is healthy, it takes the food we feed it and turns that nutrition into energy, keeping us going all day. But as the physical body weakens, its energy production decreases.

"I like to call these Energy Units," she said. "Each day when you wake up, you have a bank of Energy Units, and everything you do uses a portion of them."

"That makes sense," Mom said.

"The key to a good quality of life right now," Peggy said, "is to conserve your Energy Units. Believe it or not, even when you talk on the phone you are using energy. As an example, there may come a time when you'll decide that you'd rather watch TV or talk to your daughter, instead of reading the newspaper."

"Hmm," Mom said, contemplating that.

"I know it might sound funny," Peggy said to me, "but I suggest you buy a baby monitor as a simple way to conserve your mom's energy. If you need help," she said to Mom, "you could yell or ring a bell, but those acts would use more Energy Units than if there were a monitor in your room, right next to your bed. No matter where your daughter is in the house, she'll always be able to hear you, even if you whisper—provided she has the receiver with her."

Mom like the proposal, so I drove to Radio Shack that day and learned that the baby monitor which I called an Adult Monitor, was a great idea. We placed Mom's end of the monitor on her nightstand, and I would hook the receiver on my jeans each day, or put it in the pocket of my robe. Then, if Mom woke up, I could hear her say, *"Hi honey."* If I was downstairs, and she wanted something else, she could quietly say, *"Honey, could you bring me a glass of milk?"* and I could easily hear her. That monitor helped both of us; it saved Mom Energy Units, and it saved me multiple trips up and down the stairs.

Before leaving, Peggy took me aside. "Your mother needs someone to watch her while you're at the office. She shouldn't be left alone unless it's just for you to take a short trip to the grocery store. It's also time to bring in a portable commode, which she can place near the bed. She's using too much energy walking to the bathroom. Her energy would be better used doing things she enjoys."

"Okay," I conceded. "Thank you for telling me."

As I walked her to the door, I told her that I didn't have family or friends who were able to come stay with Mom while I worked. "Can hospice help more?" I asked.

"They'll provide nurses like me to monitor your mom," Peggy said, "and we can arrange a home health aide to bathe her. But we don't provide the caregivers."

"Okay," I sighed. "I'll try to find someone to come in while I'm away. Do you have any suggestions where I should start to look?"

"Of course," she said with a smile. "I can even give you a list of agencies, although we can't recommend one over the other. I'll fax a list over in a little bit." As she stepped out the door, she added, "I'm sure you'll find someone. And thanks for understanding that your mom is too weak to be alone."

The idea of leaving Mom with a stranger in my house turned my stomach, but I had no other choice. Trying to find additional help was not easy. In the beginning I didn't know what questions to ask. I soon learned that most agencies charged a four-hour minimum, even if the aide was only needed for two hours. I also learned that it was more expensive to hire a nurse than a home health aide. Luckily, we could get by with an aide until Mom needed someone to administer prescription medications, or if dressings needed to be changed.

I had hoped to find just one person to care for Mom, someone she could get to know and trust. But I learned that agencies couldn't guarantee that one specific person would be available each time I needed them. That was disappointing. But since it wasn't safe for her to be alone, and I didn't want her to fall or to be injured, I hired a home health aide to come stay with Mom for eight hours. She would start the first workday after Christmas.

The portable toilet arrived later in the day. It looked like a white plastic bucket covered with a toilet seat and a lid, sitting a few inches off the ground in a four-legged plastic stand. The apparatus was lightweight and easy to move, and if the lid was down I could use it as a stool. It took a period of adjustment, but we both grew to appreciate its convenience. When she needed to use the bathroom, I would hold Mom's outstretched hands and gently pull her forward into a full sitting position. After she stopped coughing, I would pull back the covers and help her swing her legs off the bed. She would lean on me as I held her elbow and arm, and I would steady her as she shuffled to sit on the potty. If she was cold, I would place my robe around her shoulders, make sure the toilet paper was nearby, and leave her alone with the television or radio playing. Once finished, she would call me back and we would reverse the process.

While she rested back in bed, I would remove the bucket, dispose of the contents in her bathroom toilet, and carry it downstairs to the kitchen sink for cleaning. Once washed and dried, I returned the bucket and moved the chair out of the way. It was simple, but as with other routines, the first time was a bit clumsy. With each passing day, however, we became more proficient and thankful to be saving Energy Units.

Thirty-nine
Mom's Tears

A t this point Mom added a new ritual, one I didn't like at all.

"Thanks so much for taking care of me honey, but I'm tired and ready to go be with your Dad. I know you'll be okay without me. I'm sorry I'm such a burden to you. Please know I love you. I just want to die in my sleep tonight, okay?"

I would tell Mom how much I loved her, and that it was okay with me if she was ready to die. I would thank her for my life and her love and guidance. Then I would turn out her light and walk down the hall with a heavy heart.

The mornings were even worse. Each day she woke up, she would burst into tears, mad that she was not in heaven with Dad. She hated waking up alone in bed. She was used to sleeping next to her husband, as she had for over fifty-two years. It was heartbreaking for me to see Mom cry, and to be honest, it hurt my feelings. I thought part of her should have been happy to still be with me.

Because I didn't know what to do, each morning after her tears we would talk, and I would assure her that I was committed to her care, that she was not a burden, that she would be doing the same thing if I were the sick one, and that I loved—absolutely loved—having her in my house. This pattern of her wanting to die each night, and then crying each morning, repeated itself for ten days. I had no idea how to make things better.

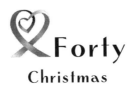

Forty

Christmas

Christmas day was certainly different than years past. Mom woke up, cried in anger, and again we talked. Eventually we read the newspaper together while savoring our morning coffee. I sat in a chair next to Mom, with Mischief lying beside her right leg. Choosing to focus on the positive, we both agreed it was a good day because I could stay home with her.

After reading the newspaper, I tied red and green ribbons around the kittens' necks, and then we played one of their favorite games. I'd throw their red plastic balls into Mom's room, and we would laugh and smile as they chased after them. They looked so cute and brought us a bit of Christmas cheer.

Mom had received over fifty Christmas cards in the prior weeks. She read through each one again, telling me who it was from, and how she knew that person. The Green Onion ladies had mailed her a Christmas gift, which we saved to open that afternoon. Inside the wrapped cardboard box was a stuffed animal, a two-foot tall brown bear, wearing a hooded red knit jacket. On his chest was a red heart. He was a cute, fuzzy invitation to hug. Mom loved that bear and I cherished Mom's friends for loving and missing her.

The phone rang at least a dozen times that day, friends and family calling for Mom. We made a few calls of our own, starting with one to check on Grandma, pleased to hear she was well. Later in the day we talked about how things could be worse. We agreed it would be harder on Mom if I were the one dying of cancer and she were taking care of me. After all, it was nature's way that a mother should die first.

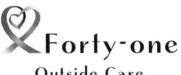

Forty-one
Outside Care
December 28

The Monday after Christmas, an agency sent a home health aide to stay with Mom for the eight hours I was at work. Before leaving for the office, I explained she was to provide assistance to Mom, giving her anything she wanted. This was the first time that the aide and Mom had been together.

Since Mom wasn't in the habit of accepting outside care, and the aide didn't want to intrude, the situation didn't appear to benefit Mom. Later that evening, Mom told me she thought paying for the aide to sit downstairs and watch TV all day was a waste of money. As with any new relationship, communication between both parties is essential, so I suggested that she should be more vocal so that the aide coming on Tuesday would better understand what she needed.

Before leaving the office Tuesday, my colleagues and I discussed my desire to find a person to care for Mom while I worked in the office. Ideally I wanted one specific person for Mom to bond with, someone I could trust and depend on. My colleagues agreed to keep their ears open for someone who might be interested in part-time work.

That Tuesday night when I came home, Mom was depressed and again the aide didn't seem to have done much more than sit downstairs and watch TV. We had different aides scheduled for Thursday and Friday, but not knowing how to resolve the communication problem, I decided to cancel those aides and instead work from home for the rest of the week.

By Friday night, I was tired and despondent. Mom had continued to decline, sleeping more and slowly slipping away. I was constantly thinking about her when I was at the office, and I debated whether to seek a leave of absence until she passed.

I walked down the stairs and sat on the last step. The kittens ran down to sit by me, hoping that I was going to play with them. Instead, with my elbows on my knees, I put my face in my hands and burst into tears, hoping that Mom couldn't hear me.

About that time, the doorbell rang. I was surprised to see Carolyn at the door. I wondered if my colleague had asked his wife to drop off some work, since neither had ever been to my house.

"Hi Carolyn, how nice to see you," I said, wiping away my tears. "May I help you with something?"

"Oh no," she replied. "Dick mentioned things are difficult with your mom, and since I was on my way home from a late-afternoon movie, I decided to stop by and say hi. I hope I'm not interrupting you. Have you been crying? Is something wrong?"

"Yes," I blurted out, without hesitating. "Mom is so much worse. She seems sad most of the time, she sleeps a lot, and I'm so scared I'm losing her. I haven't been able to find outside care that I like, and I'm frustrated. I promised her I'd take care of her—and I will—but I just don't know how. Maybe I should stop working, and stay home with her until she dies."

I quickly added, "Oh Carolyn, I'm sorry to unload and complain. It's so nice of you to stop by."

"I can't imagine how difficult this must be for you," said Carolyn, "losing your dad and now your mom. It's good to cry, to let out your emotions." I smiled as her words calmed me.

"Besides wanting to say hello, I stopped in to see if you might be interested in hiring a male nurse, who is a friend of mine."

"A male nurse?" I said, a note of surprise in my voice. "I don't know how Mom would feel about that. To be honest, I don't know how I feel about a male nurse being with Mom."

"Well," explained Carolyn, "Dick mentioned you're looking for part-time help, and I have a friend named Warren who just graduated from nursing school. He's applied to several hospitals and is waiting for his applications to be processed. I hope you don't mind, but I talked to him to see if he would be interested in helping you out a few days a week, until he's hired, and he said yes. Why don't you think about it and let me know?"

"Warren," I said, "hmmm, that name sounds familiar. Do I know him? Is that the Warren I met when we hiked with you in October?"

"Yep, that's right, you met him on the hike. He's a very reliable man, someone you could trust one hundred percent."

"Oh Carolyn, Warren would be great," I gushed. "I love the idea. Thank you so much! Let me talk with Mom, and I'll let you know. Maybe we could have him come over to meet her, before we agree to hire him. They could see if their personalities fit. What do you think?"

"I think that would be perfect," replied Carolyn. "If your mom agrees, call me and I'll call Warren. Now give me another hug," she whispered, "and know that you and your mom are in our prayers.

I felt better knowing it might work, but I wasn't sure how comfortable Mom would be with a male nurse. The only way to find out would be to suggest it and see how she responded. I decided to wait a few days, however, and planned to discuss it on a day when she felt a little better.

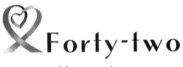

Forty-two

Honesty
December 29

Peggy was coming to see Mom. Before she arrived, I asked Mom to be honest with her, to tell her how sad she was and how she cried every morning.

It was always good to see Peggy. She was now in the habit of sitting on the bed next to Mom while I sat in the chair next to the picture window. Mom told her how angry and sad she was every morning, explaining that she would awaken disappointed to still be alive, that she was ready to die. Peggy asked if she could have some time alone with Mom and I agreed. A little later, Peggy asked me to come back.

The three of us visited for another ten minutes, talking about the news of the day, including the pending impeachment proceedings against President Clinton. Before she left, Peggy asked Mom if she was in pain. She asked her to rate it on a scale of one to ten, with one being the least bit of pain, and ten being the worst.

"*Three*," she responded.

"I appreciate your honesty. Many patients don't want to admit they're in pain, so it's hard for us to do our job and keep someone comfortable if we can't be certain how they're feeling. It would be best if we could start your treatment now — your quality of life will be much better if we stay ahead of the pain, not behind it."

"I think you would be more relaxed if we started you on morphine. In the proper dose, morphine is highly effective. Once it's in your system, if taken as suggested, it should eliminate your pain without making you groggy. It should greatly enhance your quality of life. Pain causes your body to be stressed and a stressed body uses Energy Units to fight the pain. If your body is pain free, those Energy Units may be used for other things you enjoy."

I thought that Peggy's explanation made sense, but when Peggy asked Mom if she would agree to take the morphine, Mom said no; she was adamantly against it.

As I walked Peggy down the stairs and out the door, she said that she thought Mom's quality of life would be enhanced if we could get control of her pain. She told me that the longer we waited, the harder it would be to get it under control, and so if Mom changed her mind, I should call hospice and they would send out the medicine. Peggy would order liquid morphine that I would be able to measure with a small syringe, drop the tasteless liquid into a glass, and add it to any juice. Mom wouldn't know it was even there. I guess we could have tricked her, but that was not the way of hospice. Whether or not Mom would take morphine was her decision. She was the patient, and as long as she could make choices, the decisions were hers to make.

I was surprised to learn Mom was in pain, and I wondered how long she had been hurting. I don't think even Peggy would have known if I hadn't asked Mom to be honest during this visit. Mom had been masking some of her emotions during the past two hospice visits. Maybe she had been suffering for some time.

I walked back up the stairs and into Mom's room, hoping to understand why she didn't want the morphine. "Mom, thanks for telling Peggy that you're having some pain."

"It isn't bad; nothing I can't handle."

"I'm glad the pain isn't bad, but it would be better if we could start controlling it now. You'd feel a lot better."

"Well, it really isn't bad yet. So let's just forget it for now."

"Okay," I said reluctantly, "but will you tell me why you don't want to take the morphine?"

"I don't want shots! I had to have shots ten days in a row after each chemo treatment. I didn't like them and I don't want any shots now," she shouted.

"Shots? Why do you think the morphine is given to you by a shot?"

"I've seen it at the movies. I remember people taking morphine that way."

"Mom, I believe you're thinking of heroin. You may have seen movies with people shooting heroin into their veins. The morphine Peggy wants you to take comes in liquid form. I'd be able to pour just a little bit into a glass with your juice. You could watch me do it. According to Peggy, you won't even be able to taste it. In fact, I could put it in your juice, and you wouldn't even know it was there; but this is your body, and your journey, and your choice. I'm sorry we didn't make it clearer to you, but you don't have to have shots to control your pain Mom—just liquid."

"Really? *I wouldn't need to have a shot?*" she said surprised. *"Okay, if I can drink it in my juice, let's give it a try."*

I was so relieved that I nearly burst into tears, but I didn't. Instead, I picked up the phone in Mom's room and called Peggy. I told her that Mom had agreed to try the morphine. Peggy was pleased and asked to talk with Mom for a moment. After confirming Mom's desire, Peggy said she would call in the order, and that we should expect it in a few hours. She told me to follow the instructions and give it to Mom right away. I agreed, and thanked her again. Mom said she was going to read for a while, so I left her alone, and soon she was fast asleep.

The doorbell rang a few hours later. Before I could get to the front door, the kittens ran past me, and were waiting for me to open the door to see who was coming to visit us and maybe pet them.

When I opened the front door, I saw a young man in his early twenties holding a small white paper bag that was stapled shut. I reached for the bag, but first I had to sign a form. I learned that because morphine is a controlled substance, it is strictly monitored. The state requires every pharmacy dispensing it to maintain a record with the names and signatures of every recipient. I signed the form and thanked him, again noting with pleasure there was no charge.

I walked up to Mom's room, holding the bag and a drinking glass in one hand, and a jar of cranberry juice in the other. Mom was awake, curious to see how the process worked. Inside the stapled bag was a purple glass bottle (its shape reminded me of a bottle of milk of magnesia) with two small plastic syringes. I held the bottle, twisted open the lid, inserted the syringe into the clear liquid, and pulled back slightly on the tip until I had the right dose of medicine.

Both Mom and I were skeptical that such a small amount of liquid would ease her pain. Holding the syringe with my left hand, I poured the cranberry juice into her glass. With Mom's consent, I released the tiny bit of liquid into the juice, then handed Mom the glass. Cautiously she took a sip, pleased to discover she could only taste the cranberry juice. She looked at me and took another sip. Apparently Peggy was right; Mom couldn't taste the morphine. She finished the juice, and we sat and waited.

We both thought that she would feel the morphine right away, similar to the way you feel the first sip of a good martini. But for Mom, that wasn't the way it worked. In fact, I am not sure Mom even noticed her pain easing away.

What we did notice was that as the days passed, Mom started to enjoy life again. She wasn't tired or grouchy all the time; she felt like reading again and was sleeping less. It was an amazing reversal, and for the next six weeks it was as though time had been turned back. The best news was that she stopped wanting to die at night and didn't cry when she woke in the morning.

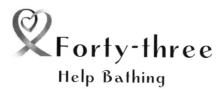

Forty-three
Help Bathing

When Mom was too weak to walk to the shower, we tried to keep her clean with washcloth baths, the type she used to give me when I was a child with a fever. The first time we tried it, it was okay, but it still tired her because she tried to do most of the work. I tried to help more the second time, but I probably made it worse, soaking both Mom and the bed.

Mom and I revisited Peggy's offer to send an aide to bathe her in bed, assuming they knew how to do it better than we did. If someone else was doing the work, then Mom could conserve her Energy Units.

On the first day of January, Mom and I told Peggy that we would agree to hospice sending someone to bathe her. Peggy suggested we schedule a bed bath twice a week. We had no idea what would be appropriate, so we agreed.

We were nervous because it could be an embarrassing time for Mom; but more than that, we were curious to learn the proper way to manage the process. Once again, we were lucky, and right away we both liked the hospice home health aide, Janice. She was kind, caring, and very considerate. She liked to talk, listen, and laugh, which made Mom very happy.

It was amazing, but Janice gave Mom a full bath. She even washed Mom's hair with a shampoo that didn't need to be rinsed. Afterwards, she changed Mom's clothes, and then she gently blew dry her hair and brushed her teeth. If that wasn't enough of a welcome surprise, she filed Mom's nails and rubbed lotion on her arms, legs, hands, and feet. While Mom was being cared for, they visited. When Janice left, Mom felt fresh and clean. As the weeks passed, the two bonded, and Mom always looked forward to her visits.

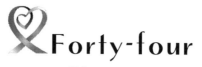

Forty-four
Warren
January 7, 1999

For the past few days Mom had been feeling better. I believe it was a combination of the morphine eliminating her pain, using fewer Energy Units, enjoying Janice, and my working from home.

I was so happy that Mom was feeling better, but I had learned that because she was taking morphine only a licensed nurse, not an aide, could dispense the morphine. I decided it was a good time to talk about her meeting with the male nurse to help when I was working at the office.

"Mom, Dick's wife, Carolyn, has a friend, a recent nursing school graduate, whose applications are being processed at several hospitals. He's willing to come take care of you part-time. Would you mind if I called to set up a meeting between the two of you?"

"No, I don't mind. I know that it's hard on you, worrying about me while you're working. So if it's someone you like and trust, have her come over."

"Um, Mom," I stuttered, "the nurse is not a she, it's a he."

"A male nurse? I don't think so honey. You know I don't have the energy to walk to the bathroom, and I have to use that portable potty. That would be embarrassing having a male nurse helping me."

"I know, Mom," I said with empathy. "I can understand how you feel. It just would be so nice to have one other person caring for you besides me, someone we can rely upon and trust."

She wasn't yet convinced.

"Oh, I forgot to tell you--I know him too — or at least I've met him. Remember when I went hiking with Carolyn in October, and I told you about the people I met? He was the gentleman wearing the Costco socks. He recently graduated from nursing school."

"Oh, yes. I remember the guy you said was wearing the Costco socks. You said you liked him. If you liked him, maybe I would too. I guess if I was in a hospital I would probably have male nurses, wouldn't I?" I nodded.

"Mom, what if he came over to talk with you? If you don't like him, then we won't hire him."

"Okay, I know it will make you feel better, so I'll meet him."

Warren arrived the next day. He was well dressed, wearing tan slacks, a pressed shirt, and polished shoes. I brought him upstairs to Mom's room, first making sure that he wasn't allergic to the kittens. I introduced Warren to Mom and stayed a little while, then excused myself and left the room. Warren talked with Mom for about forty-five minutes. I walked him downstairs, thanked him for coming over right away, and told him I would call him with an update.

After saying good-bye, I ran upstairs to Mom's room, eager to hear her thoughts, but nervous at the same time. "Well Mom, what did you think about Warren?"

"I think we should give him a try. He seems nice and he is a nurse so if something was wrong he could help me. I showed him our picture and told him all about Dad. Can we try him out and if it doesn't work change our mind?"

"Of course we can," I sighed with relief. We hired Warren that very day and he worked out even better than we expected.

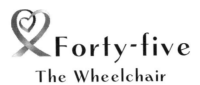

Forty-five
The Wheelchair

Our next change was the introduction of the wheelchair that was delivered to our front door and carried upstairs, once again at no charge to us. The wheelchair helped when it was time for me to change Mom's sheets, which I liked to do every three or four days.

I would roll the wheelchair to the side of Mom's bed, and help her put on her robe and slippers. Then I would lift her off the bed and place her into the wheelchair. I'd then take her into my bedroom, kittens in tow, where she could look out the window. Across Warrenson Bay was the Bothin Marsh Preserve, where twice she had seen a Great Egret fly by, and she was constantly on the lookout for others.

On my way back to her room, I opened the hall closet, grabbing fresh yellow sheets. Every time I changed her sheets, I would wonder if this would be the last time. Such thoughts were impossible to stop and I would change the linens slowly, performing the task with extra care. Like my trips to the grocery store, this was my quiet time and I knew Mom enjoyed the change of scenery.

Sometimes Mischief would run into the room after I had thrown the comforter on the floor, and jump onto the bed wanting to play. I would cover her with the sheets; she would roll around, searching for a way out. Finding an opening, she would dart out, jump off the bed, and fly out of the room.Ten seconds later she would return, diving once again into the sheets, hoping we could play a bit more. She thought it was a game just for her, and since it made me laugh and prolonged my quiet time, I joined in her fun. After a few more runs, she would stop, falling over to rest on the carpet near the bedroom door, tired but still wanting to be close.

The clean sheets, plumped pillows, and turned-down bedspread always made Mom's bed appear neat and inviting. I would then walk back into my room, and if Mom was feeling okay, I might sit on the edge of my bed and chat with her about the weather, the scenery, or the news. Eventually I would wheel her back to her bedroom, where the smell of fresh sheets invited us in. Once she was comfortably settled in the bed, she would sigh in delight, and for the moment our world was better.

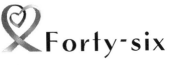

Forty-six

January 10, 1999

That Sunday was one of our better days. For the first time in a month, Mom asked me to cook her breakfast. She wanted one crisp piece of bacon, a fried egg, and an English muffin with strawberry jam. With joy, I cooked and carried her breakfast upstairs. She ate every bite and drank a full glass of milk!

The hospice nurse had told us that the morphine might make Mom feel better, and she was right. Two weeks prior she had been depressed, sleeping most of the day and feeling awful. The previous month, I hadn't been sure that Mom would be alive in January, yet that day she felt good. I thought she would be with me for several more months, long enough to see the tree outside her window bloom.

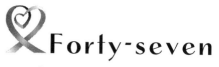

Forty-seven

Love in My Home

K nowing that Mom was in my house was a gift. She was the first person I said good morning to and the last person I kissed good night.

We settled into a new routine. I would get up each morning and drink my coffee, while I got ready for work. As I ate a bowl of cereal, I would clean out the coffee pot, then add fresh water and coffee, so it was ready to brew when Mom woke up. I would look into Mom's room several times each morning to be sure she was okay. Usually she heard me and would say good morning. If she was tired, she would go back to sleep. I would leave for the office about eight, as soon as Warren arrived. He would give me a hug as I handed him the Adult Monitor, then sit downstairs and wait for Mom to wake up. Once awake, he would brew her coffee. Then, he'd walk upstairs with a cup in hand, give Mom her medicine, hand her the newspaper, help with her morning needs, and keep her company.

I returned home each day at about 6:30 p.m. Before leaving, Warren would give me a briefing of their day together. He had the patience of a saint. I bet he looked through each page of her picture album twice daily. If Mom wanted to visit, Warren was ready to talk. If she wanted time alone, he would honor her wish.

Some days Mom felt better than others. On a good day she would read the morning *San Francisco Chronicle*, talk with friends on the phone, visit with Warren, and watch her television shows. Except for that one Sunday morning breakfast, her appetite was now nearly gone. After she had eaten her grapefruit, all she wanted for the rest of the day was Jell-O, ice cream, and one Ensure. She would also try to drink a lot of water as it helped with her bowel movements. She loved reading her mail, always interested to learn how her friends were spending their days.

At night, I would sit in a chair by Mom's bed. While we talked, I might sip a beer or glass of wine, a continuation of the cocktail hour she and Dad shared for so many years. Whether I had worked at the office or at home, we would share the events of our day. She would tell me whom she had talked to that day and read me every card she had received. She came to know many of the daily issues I faced at work, sharing her thoughts and occasionally offering solutions for me to consider. We also discussed President Clinton's impeachment proceedings, although we were careful with this issue since she was an avid Rush Limbaugh listener and I was not.

On days that Warren cared for Mom, he would arrive with a plant or magazine, always bringing her something he knew she would enjoy. Even on his days off, he would call to see how she was feeling.

Unlike most people, when I am under stress, food is not appealing. Even though I didn't have an appetite, as Mom's primary caregiver I had to stay healthy. So each night I'd sacrifice a portion of my time with her to cook something healthy. As long as the smell didn't make her nauseous, I would bring whatever I had prepared upstairs and eat it in the chair next to her bed.

In January, while we were watching TV, out of the corner of my eye I would notice her outstretched left hand. I would take it in my right hand, giving her a loving light squeeze while we sat together, hand in hand. Most nights our television preference was either *Seinfeld* or *Frasier*. It didn't matter if we had seen the show before; the goal was to laugh and forget, even for a moment, our reality. On Saturdays we would look forward to watching Mom's two favorite English comedies: *Mr. Bean* and *Keeping Up Appearances*. They both guaranteed laughter.

We would talk or watch TV until about 9:30, when, once again, we would begin our evening ritual. Sometimes, when I was very tired, I would impatiently think to myself, "This takes too long; hurry up, Mom; who cares if your skin is nourished tonight, or your teeth are spotless?" It took me awhile to realize that Mom's evening routine was important to her, not only because it made her feel good, but because it was one thing in her life that had not changed. When I figured that out, I became much more patient.

Before I turned out the light, we ended each evening with a good night kiss. Walking down the hall to my bedroom, with two kittens at my heels, I would say prayers of gratitude for one more day with Mom. She was well cared for, and I could check on her throughout the day. When she felt well, we could talk and laugh. Our time together was not interrupted by doctors or nurses working on timetables that required them to take her blood pressure or draw blood. At home we made our own schedule. Things were not as we wanted, but given the circumstances, they were as good as we could expect.

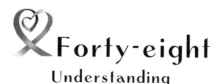

Forty-eight

Understanding

There were times, especially on days when I was tired, that Mom would tell me what to do and it would really irritate me.

"Throw those newspapers out."

"Put my telephone book away."

"Move the clock to where I can see it."

"Be sure my box of tissue is near the top of the bed so I can reach it."

"Take the papers off the throw blanket at the end of the bed so the kittens have a place to sleep."

"Hand me my box of cards."

At first I thought Mom's instructions were cute and gave her something to do. But as time passed, and I heard the same instructions day after day, her orders became annoying.

For my own sanity, I called hospice and left a message for Joe to call me. I thought he might have suggestions to help ease my frustrations. He called me back that same day and listened while I complained.

Joe helped me understand that those instructions were all Mom had left to control. At one time, she controlled her life, her husband's life, and my life. She planned what we would eat and wear and took care of us. Now she could no longer get out of bed. She could not care for her husband, for her daughter, or even for herself. She could not plan anything, even the timing of her own death.

What she could do is try to control what her surroundings looked like, to keep it neat and organized. Her bed became a miniature replication of the world she once controlled.

Thank goodness for Joe. After talking with him, Mom's instructions no longer affected me in the same manner.

Forty-nine

Planning Her Good-Byes

Beginning in January and through mid-February, we enjoyed six good weeks. Warren was a huge help. Mom enjoyed his every visit and thought of him more as a friend than a nurse.

During that time, Mom regained the energy to write checks and pay her bills. Together we planned for the future. Mom even helped me draft her obituary.

"I want my obituary to say that I died of lung cancer."

Sometimes I couldn't help myself, and the factual attorney in me would emerge.

"But Mom, you don't have lung cancer. Technically, what you have is uterine cancer that has metastasized to your lungs. It isn't lung cancer, even though it probably feels like lung cancer."

"I don't care what it is. It's cancer. Right now it's in my lungs. Your father died of lung cancer, and I want my obituary to read the same as his."

"Okay Mom, then that's what it will say."

We also spent time trying to decide whether I should have a memorial for Mom. We both knew that most of the people who came to Dad's memorial would be the same ones invited to Mom's service.

We both also knew that I hadn't yet grieved for Dad. After Mom died I would need down time to rest and grieve for both of them. Would I be ready to travel to Southern California right away and coordinate another memorial?

We talked about it for several nights. She decided to make a list with the names of friends that she would want me to call after she left us. She agreed that if I felt like it, I could invite those people on her list, but if I didn't think I could handle another memorial that was fine with her. I promised Mom I would call each of her friends after she died.

For the next few evenings, after I came home from work, she would show me her growing list. She would spend time each day reviewing every name in her address book. Not only did she write down the name of each person she wanted me to call, she also had included their address and phone number. If I didn't know the person, she included an identifier reminding me how or when she met them, such as "my friend in third grade," or "worked with at the bank in Whittier," or "met on a Caribbean cruise."

In addition, she made another list of things I was supposed to tell her friends. I was to say thanks to everyone who continued to call. She wanted me to tell Constance how much she admired her courage and poise when her daughter died at age fourteen; I was to tell Earl and Dick how much it meant that they called and sent letters after they learned Dad died, even though she had not talked to them for nearly twenty years. Mom wanted me to tell Harvey, the best man at their wedding, that she never forgot the day Dad proposed in Harvey's car—Dad and Mom in the back seat, Harvey sitting behind the wheel. I was to tell Annabelle how much Mom admired her laughter during the years when Annabelle didn't have any reason to smile.

She wanted me to thank her friends and neighbors in Palm Desert (including the Green Onion Ladies) for making Dad and her life so wonderful during their retirement. She wanted me to thank her in-laws for giving her a second family. I was to tell her friends from Santa Barbara that she never forgot them. She wanted me to thank Norma for always being available and to remind Issy she loved her.

She wanted me to ensure her mother's good care. She wanted me to remember how she and Dad loved me, and she wanted me to have more confidence.

I had jobs to do after she departed.

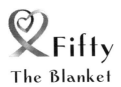

Fifty

The Blanket

B efore Mom came to live with me, I was just one of many anonymous customers on my postman's route. In late November, anticipating her move, we had forwarded her mail to my address, thus substantially increasing my daily mail.

One day, I was outside watering the plants when the postman arrived. We introduced ourselves, and he politely asked why I received so much mail addressed to my Mom. I explained she had a life-limiting illness, that she had lived in Southern California, that my Father had recently died, and that she moved in so I could take care of her. He told me it was rare for him to deliver so much mail addressed to one person on a daily basis.

During our "Last Months" Mom received over two hundred cards from friends and family. As the cards grew in number, the box she stored them in changed in size. That box was either on her bed or next to it, and she read each card several times a week. The cards connected her with her past and confirmed she was remembered and loved.

In late January our postman delivered a box addressed to Mom that was about eight inches high and two feet long. As I carried it upstairs, I thought it would be the perfect box for her cards.According to

179

the return address, it was from Mom's high school friend, Annabelle. We were both excited to learn what was in the box, so I ran downstairs to get the scissors.

By the time I came back upstairs, both kittens were on the bed with Mom, sniffing the new addition. I used the scissors to open the box, and then Mom ripped open the tissue covering the contents. Inside was a folded blue and cream-colored throw blanket. Mom read the words "Surf City" on one part of the blanket; next, "oil wells"; then "July 4th parade"; and finally, "Huntington Beach pier."

Those last words caused Mom to burst into tears. She must have sobbed for five minutes. The kittens, who had been sharing the moment, took off running, and I wished I could have followed them. I didn't know what to do. I wanted to stuff the blanket back into the box and pretend like we never saw it. More tears—just what we needed!

Eventually Mom dried her eyes. *"Honey, these aren't sad tears, they're tears of joy. I loved both my life in Huntington Beach and my friend, Annabelle. Those were my happy days with my mom and dad. I was so lucky to live in Huntington Beach, a small town where we all knew each other. Mom and Dad were happy because Daddy finally had a secure job. I had fun for four years at a wonderful high school with my dear friends. Life was simple. The big bands played, I could go to Catalina Island for dances, and I met your Dad. It was a wonderful time in my life. I love this blanket. Look, here's Huntington Beach High School, too! What a wonderful gift. Would you hand me the phone so I can call Annabelle and thank her?"*

I still have that blanket and the cardboard box, filled with all the cards she received. Both were tucked away in my closet for years, too dear a reminder of Mom for me to have out, and too precious to throw away. The cards are still in the closet, but not the blanket.

The Huntington Beach Historical Society's blue and cream blanket, celebrating Huntington Beach's 1888-1998 Centennial, is proudly draped across my couch. Mom loved that blanket, and so do I.

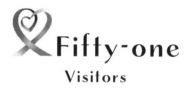

Fifty-one

Visitors

In January, Mom enjoyed three visits from loved ones who drove north from Los Angeles to say their good-byes.

Mom looked forward to all three visits. We scheduled her bed baths for the day before her guests arrived, and I made sure her sheets were clean and her bedroom was neat. An hour before each arrival, Mom would carefully apply her make-up and brush her hair. She was happy to see those she loved, people with whom she had shared so much of her life.

For me, the visits were a mixed blessing. On the one hand, I loved Mom looking forward to the visits; it was wonderful to see family, and I too enjoyed having someone else in the house. On the other hand, I was the caregiver, the worker, and also the house cleaner. For me the visits meant additional work before each visit and sorrow after. Before our guests arrived, I gave up sleep to vacuum, dust, clean floors and sinks, tidy Mom's room, and make an extra trip to the grocery store to buy snacks and drinks.

It didn't seem to bother Mom that she had to entertain in the bedroom. I would bring chairs up from the dining room, so that Mom could be close to each guest.

Each visit followed the same pattern: the doorbell would ring, the cats would run downstairs hoping to get petted, and I would open the door and receive a long hug.

In my dining room we would talk in low tones as I explained that Mom was doing much better than a few weeks ago. I didn't share the stress of being a caregiver, the grief I was carrying over the loss of Dad, or the pain in my heart knowing I would soon be losing Mom. I acted like working full-time and caring for her was easy, not wanting to distract from their visit. I knew only too well that focusing on saying good-bye needed their full attention.

I would thank them for coming, and then lead them upstairs into her room. After making sure everyone had a place to sit, a glass of juice, and a snack, I would leave them alone to talk. If it wasn't raining, I would get out of the house and walk for a few miles, thinking about how life had changed. We used to have visitors at least once a month; we would talk, eat, laugh, and plan the next get together. Now they were saying good-bye. I knew it would soon be my turn to say good-bye, but I still wasn't ready.

Once back home, I would sit downstairs until I heard someone call my name, then bound upstairs. Sometimes I could tell that tears had been shed, although I never asked. I considered each visit a private matter, and so did Mom. After our visitors had left, I would return upstairs to see how she was doing. In the few minutes I'd been gone, her smiling, positive, and thankful mood was replaced by a sad, pensive one. Soon she was sound asleep, exhausted by the emotions of the day.

In the quiet house, with Mom worn out, I would sit in silence, devastated that my best friend would soon be gone, leaving me alone. I would slowly clean up the kitchen, feeling sorry for myself, tired of preparing for guests and selfishly wanting all her time. Caregiving is not for the weak of heart.

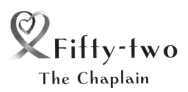

Fifty-two

The Chaplain

One of the many services that hospice offered us was the opportunity to have a chaplain visit whenever we wanted. I had yet to join a church in the area and Mom had not regularly attended church in the desert. Although we weren't members of a specific church, both of us wanted to talk with a minister.

The chaplain hospice sent to visit with us was named Gay. She was about my age, and we both found her to be caring and comforting. She came to our house on five separate occasions.

On her first visit, she met with us and listened as Mom told her life story, politely looking through Mom's picture book. We immediately knew we had a new friend, one we enjoyed having in the house.

On her second visit, Gay stayed more than an hour, visiting only with Mom. Mom may have asked her what to expect when she died; I don't know. Mom never discussed her visits with Gay, and I knew their time together was intimate.

On her third and forth visits, I needed and shared part of Gay's time. I listened to her read from the bible and watched as she blessed Mom and anointed her with sacred oil.

Mom and I viewed the fact that Gay came to see us several times as an honor and we treated her with the respect she deserved.

She brought peace and calm to our home, and each time she left I was surrounded by a feeling that my future would be okay.

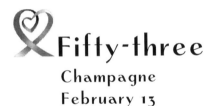

Fifty-three

Champagne
February 13

Throughout Mom's illness, both my boss and my work colleagues were extremely supportive. Together they thought of a unique way to help us celebrate Valentine's Day. This was not going to be the best one Mom and I had ever shared, because although she had received many cards, it was not the same without Dad. We had not intended to celebrate, but things changed when we received the card and the bottle of champagne from my office. How could we turn down a special gift of the bubbly, given with love? And it wasn't just any brand; my colleagues surprised us with a bottle of Dom Perignon.

Neither Mom nor I had ever sipped Dom Perignon, so since it was a gift, we agreed to enjoy a taste on Saturday, the evening before Valentine's Day. That night, while the rest of the world was out celebrating Valentine's Day, Mom and I had our own private celebration.

We waited until Mom's favorite British television show, *Keeping Up Appearances*, came on. As the program started by showing a fancy dinner table set with an eight-piece candelabra, we thought that was a fitting way to start our evening with champagne. Mom had slept well that afternoon and felt pretty good all evening.

I brought the chilled champagne and two glasses up to Mom's room. I was very careful not to spill a drop as I poured Mom half a glass and myself a full one.

"I love you Mom," I toasted. "Here's to you. Thank you for being my special Valentine."

"*I love you too honey. I know you'll be okay after I'm gone. You have lots of friends who love you and will take care of you. Thank you so much for taking care of me.*"

We clinked our glasses and had a sip. Wow, Dom Perignon didn't taste like the champagne we were used to drinking. It was a real treat, something we knew Dad would have loved.

"Here's to you, Dad, the best husband and father in the world."

We clinked our glasses again and enjoyed another sip. For the next hour, Mom and I laughed and enjoyed remembering their lives together.

"*Honey, I have had a perfect life. I loved living in Huntington Beach. My parents were loving, kind, and fun. I fell in love with your Dad, and lived fifty-two years as his devoted wife. We saw so many places together. We traveled to New York City; we marveled at the fall colors on the East Coast; we enjoyed Hawaii, and cruises to Alaska, the Caribbean, Sweden, Norway, and Russia. We saw London, and toured through many parts of Europe. We raised a wonderful daughter. I lived when Ronald Reagan was president, when Frank Sinatra was king; and got to dance during the Big Band era. And the movies; oh, they were so wonderful, years ago. I've been so very lucky, loving every day of my life, loving your Dad and loving you.*"

"I want you to love every day of your life as well. That is one of life's secrets. Enjoy what God gives you; be kind and respect others. Keep your friends and have fun making new ones--they will take care of you after I'm gone."

I wanted that wonderful, unforgettable evening with Mom to last forever. I knew Mom was dying but I didn't want to let her go. I loved her so very much, how would I live without her?

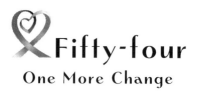

Fifty-four
One More Change

By the middle of February, things were going as well as could be expected. Mom was sleeping a little more, but she wasn't in pain. She had the energy to talk on the phone and visit with me after work. She still loved reading the newspaper from front to back, and each day she would read through the many cards she had received.

One evening after work during our de-briefing, Warren told me he received the job offer he had been waiting for. He would only be able to work for us for one more week. I was devastated. Our arrangement had been working so well. How could this be? Where was I going to find more help?

Before we hired him, Warren had warned us that he had applied for a nursing position at a hospital, and that if he were offered the position, he would accept it. He had been a gift in our lives. Because we liked him we didn't want him to leave; it was also because we liked him that we wanted what was best for Warren. So I congratulated him and wished him well. I thanked him for the love and care he had given to Mom, and I tried not to let him know how crushed I was.

Warren could see I was upset. He said he would make some calls that evening to see if other nurses he knew would have time to help us.

I hated to tell Mom that Warren would be leaving us. When I did tell her, I could see that she was even more disappointed than I was. She had grown attached to Warren, and now she was faced with another loss.

Once again we were very fortunate. Warren found another nurse from his class who would be able to help us. Her name was Julie; she had two children in middle school, but she was willing to find after-school care for them two days a week if that would help us.

Julie came to meet us a few days later. She was younger and taller than I, but a little older than Warren. She was attractive, with dark hair, wearing soft pink nursing scrubs. After introducing her to Mom, I stayed and visited for a few minutes before leaving them to get acquainted. Once Julie had left, I dashed back up to Mom's bedroom to hear her thoughts.

"I like her very much. How nice of Warren to find her for us."

Julie was one more blessing on our journey. It turned out that she was the perfect nurse for those last difficult weeks, spending every Tuesday and Thursday getting to know and care for Mom. Although Mom was sleeping more, she still had the energy to show Julie her picture album, share her life story, and ask Julie about her family.

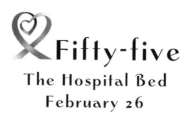

Fifty-five
The Hospital Bed
February 26

Friday turned out to be a big day for us. I had worked at the office Thursday, and now I was home—Mom's sole caregiver until Julie came again the following Tuesday.

Work was stressful and home was stressful. I was tired, I was scared to lose Mom, and I was irritable.

My back was aching more and more each day, making it physically hard for me to do the lifting required for Mom's daily care. Each time she needed to use the portable commode, she needed to be lifted up and positioned with her feet near the edge of the bed, lifted again onto the commode, and then the process was reversed to get her back into bed.

It was harder and harder for me to lift her up at night during our evening ritual. For two months Mom had refused a hospital bed. I thought she was refusing it because Dad had refused one. I also believe it was because in our minds a hospital bed meant that she was one step closer to dying. It's unfortunate we didn't realize earlier the comfort that bed would provide.

Just before noon that Friday morning, I sat on the edge of Mom's bed. Even with Advil my back still hurt. I was afraid that much more lifting might cause serious injury, and then I wouldn't be able to care for

192

Mom. She might have to leave my house, and then we wouldn't reach our goal.

"Mom, what would you think about getting you a hospital bed? It's getting harder and harder for me to lift you out of bed. I don't want to hurt myself, because then I wouldn't be able to care for you. I know you're enjoying this bed, but selfishly I need you to consider accepting a hospital bed. Do you remember when Peggy told us that the hospital bed would make it easier for you to lift yourself and that she thought it would be much more comfortable for you? Well, I really think it's time. Maybe if we ask for it today we can have it by next week. What do you think?"

"Okay honey, I didn't realize that your back was hurting you so much. I'm so sorry. If you think it will be easier for you, then go ahead and order the bed."

"Mom, thanks so much for listening, and for understanding."

I leaned over and gave Mom a hug and a kiss. I called hospice, and explained that our nurse Peggy had been suggesting we get a hospital bed and that we were now ready to order one.

"Good," the lady on the phone said. "You'll be pleased with the bed. We can have it delivered to your home today by three this afternoon. Is that okay? You'll need to remove the bed you're presently using, but we'll deliver the hospital bed and set it up for you."

"Today? Oh my, that's wonderful!" I gushed. "I think I can find someone to come over and move the bed we have. If I can't find help, then I'll call you back; otherwise, we'll look forward to the delivery of the other bed later today. Thank you so much!"

Mom and I looked at each other in amazement again. We felt so lucky to have heard about the incredible services that made hospice such a special organization.

I called the office, and two of my colleagues agreed to drive over around two and move the current bed into my garage. Fifteen minutes before they arrived, I dressed Mom in warmer clothes, covered her with a robe, and placed slippers on her feet. I carefully lifted her into the wheelchair.

I wheeled her into my bedroom where she could look outside and watch the people walking by. She said she was fine and that she would enjoy the view. I went back to her bedroom, stripped the bed, and did all I could to get it ready to be moved. About that time, the guys arrived. I let them in and introduced them to Mom.

They talked to her for a few minutes, making her feel like she was the queen of the ball. After they said their good-byes, I grabbed the kittens and shut them in my bedroom with Mom.

My colleagues took the bed apart and carried the heavy queen mattresses down the stairs, storing them for me in my garage. Before three they were on their way.

When I opened my bedroom door, the kittens ran out to explore what was new in Mom's room. I could see the back of Mom as she sat in her wheelchair. She looked so tiny, frail, and sick. It scared me to see her that way. Maybe seeing her in a different setting opened my eyes. This new reality made me sad to the core.

Walking back to Mom's bedroom, I wondered if I had made the right choice by insisting on the hospital bed. Without the queen-size bed, her two nightstands appeared even more cluttered. On one nightstand were Mom's Adult Monitor, syringes for measuring the morphine, bottles of pills for depression, anxiety, and constipation, a telephone, her address book, and a box of Kleenex. On the other nightstand were a glass of water, Mom's radio, her photo album, and the box of cards she cherished.

My thoughts were interrupted by the doorbell ringing. Opening the door, I was greeted by a friendly man in his fifties, ready to deliver and set up the hospital bed. He walked up the stairs to see the room.

I was surprised it didn't take him more than twenty minutes to bring in the twin hospital bed and the adjustable utility table that accompanied it, set them up, and make sure they both worked. As the deliveryman showed me how to operate the controls and how to put the bed rails up and down, I asked him if he had ever used the wonderful services of hospice.

"No," he said, "my family has been blessed with good health."

So were we, I thought, until life changed.

After he left I opened the bedroom door. Immediately the kittens ran down the hall into Mom's room to inspect the new bed.

"Mom, the bed is here and it looks comfy. Just give me a few more minutes while I put on clean sheets."

I didn't have twin sheets, but the queen sheets worked just fine, easily covering the egg crate foam three-inch mattress pad. By three thirty, Mom was back in the new bed. An hour later we knew we had made the right decision.

The new bed was much more comfortable for Mom. With the controls, she could now raise her back so that she could see TV better, and she could also raise her legs and feet for added comfort. And I could raise the side rails—no more worrying about her falling out of the bed at night.

The only ones who weren't immediately pleased with the new bed were the kittens. The noise of the bed moving scared them, but they adapted quickly and by evening, everyone was happy.

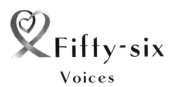

Fifty-six
Voices

L ate in February a funny thing happened. It was after dusk and Mom and I were sitting in her room. Perhaps the TV was on, I can't be sure; it could have been that we were both reading and simply enjoying each other's company. Mom had been making perfect sense all day, so I knew it didn't have anything to do with her medication.

"Did you hear that? They're talking you know."

"I didn't hear anything," I replied. "Who are you talking about, Mom?"

"Well, of course you did. They were talking in regular voices."

"Who was talking? There's no one else here, Mom."

"Didn't you see them? They were standing at the edge of my bed."

"No, I didn't see or hear anyone, Mom. Sorry."

The next evening, about the same time, Mom and I were again quietly spending time together in her room when Mom said, *"There it is again. You heard that, didn't you?"*

"Hear what Mom?"

"Well, I can't believe you didn't hear them."

"No, Mom, sorry, I didn't hear anything. Are they scaring you?"

"No, not at all. I just don't understand why you can't hear them."

Five minutes passed and Mom once again said, *"Well, you must have heard that, didn't you?"*

I had to laugh. "No Mom, I didn't hear that either. I think that's because they're here to talk to you, maybe get you ready for your journey. It's not my time to go, so they aren't here to talk to me."

She was a little angry with me because I couldn't hear them, but I think my explanation satisfied her. She never mentioned them again. I have since read that what Mom saw and heard is not uncommon. I found those two evenings very interesting, but not scary. I have often thought about those moments with her.

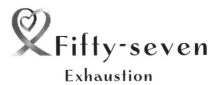

Fifty-seven
Exhaustion

By the end of February, I was exhausted; being a caregiver is physically and emotionally draining. I was sad, still reeling from the loss of Dad and not ready to let Mom go. I was also mentally exhausted from working full-time. If I was at the office, I put in a long day. If I was at home, whenever Mom was resting or didn't need me, I was at my desk, working on the computer or talking on the phone. I didn't know how I would make it through one more day. I had not anticipated that Mom would live through February. I forgot this was her timetable, and not mine.

One morning, I woke up crying from exhaustion. I knew I couldn't be much good for Mom in that condition, so not knowing where to turn, I called hospice and left a message for Joe to call me. He called right back, and three hours later he was sitting in our living room.

The fact that Joe came to our home so quickly, the fact that someone cared about me, caused me to burst into sobs. I cried tears of sorrow because Mom was going to die and tears of frustration because she had not yet died. I wanted to give her the very best care, but I was scared I wasn't doing a good enough job. I also felt I was letting down my colleagues by not being at the office every day.

Joe listened to me. He understood my fears, tears, and exhaustion and helped me understand that what I was feeling was expected and normal. He reminded me that I had several options.

Hospice offered a respite service for caregivers. If I wanted, with all costs paid by hospice, they would move Mom to a nursing home for up to five days to provide me time to rest. It was a good option, but not wanting Mom to leave my house, it didn't feel right to me at the time.

Joe suggested that I hire additional nursing care. With more help, I could sleep through the night, instead of waking every four hours to give Mom her medicine. I liked that alternative. It would be an additional expense, but well worth it. Joe and I continued to talk, and eventually I noticed that I had smiled.

I felt so much better. It was wonderful to have someone I could call who would listen to my fears, understand my journey, and provide alternative paths to help me accomplish my goal. I appreciated him more than he would ever know.

And then Joe offered a third option. "Remember," he said, "we could also send a hospice volunteer to your home to give you a break. The volunteer would sit with your Mother while you went to lunch, to a movie, or to visit with a friend. It's one of the services we've offered to you before."

I remembered, but I didn't want a hospice volunteer because I was resistant to leaving a stranger in the house with Mom. I wanted to be home with her as much as I could, partly because I was afraid that she might die while I was gone, and partly because I worried that in later years I would resent having not been with her for those few hours I was out of the house.

In hindsight, I realize that was a mistake on my part. No doubt Mom would have enjoyed meeting someone new with whom she could share her life story and learn about the person's life, and I certainly could have used the time away. Most likely, it would have resulted in my being a better, more patient caregiver. Not knowing, I just did the best I could.

♡ Fifty-eight

Julie coming two days a week worked well for me. As it became clear that Mom's body was starting to shut down, I wanted to be with her as much as possible because I knew our days together were numbered. On the two days that Julie came to be with Mom, I would go into the office. On the other days, I stayed home, working every moment I was not caring for Mom.

Each morning, before my eyes opened, I would lie in bed listening to Mom breathe through the Adult Monitor. We have another day, I would think, reaching down to pet the kittens sleeping at the end of my bed. I would get up, put on my robe and slippers, attach the receiver to my robe belt, and tiptoe down the hall to peek in on Mom. I would stand at the door to her room, comforted to see her sleeping. After a few minutes, I would tiptoe back down the hall, then walk downstairs to brew a cup of coffee. I enjoyed half and half with my coffee, which required me to open the refrigerator door, where that ever-present DNR form hung. Inside the refrigerator, the shelves were filled more with medicine bottles than with food. How our lives had changed.

After my coffee, I would force myself to eat cereal or a piece of toast with peanut butter. Once the kittens were fed and their litter box cleaned, I'd walk slowly back up the stairs.

Again I would quietly walk down to Mom's room and peek around the door frame to see if she was awake. If she was sleeping I would take my shower, then check in on her again when I had finished.

Sometimes I had to wake her so that she could take her medicine on time. I would diligently record the day, time, and medication in the notebook we kept on her nightstand. The information helped me remember what to give her next and allowed Julie and the hospice team to know what medicine had been taken and when.

Once Mom woke up, the coughing would start. I would sit by her on the bed until these persistent bouts subsided, then assist her to the portable toilet. By the time she took her medicine, used the commode, and got situated back in bed, her energy was drained. The Energy Units were now being used for just the daily necessities. Mom would still try to read the newspaper but would fall asleep within minutes.

There were days when she was so tired and weak that she would barely talk with me. The phone would ring and a friend would ask if Mom felt like talking. I would describe how bad she was feeling that day, that she was very weak and tired, but I would check to see if she would take the call. If Mom was awake, I would tell her who was on the phone and ask if she wanted to say hello. Most of the time, her answer was yes. To my amazement, she would answer in a strong voice, not her quiet, weak one that had just talked to me. I could hear her tell whoever was on the phone that she felt fine, that all was good. She would talk and laugh and tell the person how glad she was they had called and that she missed them.

Standing outside her bedroom door, listening to her talk on the phone as if she was fine, sometimes made my blood pressure rise in anger. Just moments before the phone rang she had been listless, weak, and tired; now, she was laughing, sounding fine. Her friends must have thought I was crazy, preaching doom and gloom while hearing a different story from Mom. Then Mom would finish her phone call and say good-bye, too drained to reach over and hang up the phone. Coming in to help her, I could see that she was exhausted, and in minutes she would be fast asleep.

I would think, no, I'm not crazy. Then I would get mad at her because she had just used Energy Units talking to a friend when she could have been talking to me. I was the one caring for her, putting my life on hold. I was her daughter. I needed her more than that friend on the phone. Then I would feel guilty for having those thoughts, for getting mad at her. Of course she wanted to talk with her friends; they were part of her life too. She was probably tired of just me all the time.

Next I would be sad, thinking of life without her. My anger would melt into guilt and then into sadness and tears. I rode an emotional roller coaster several times a day during those last few weeks.

Eventually Mom became too tired to talk to any of her friends. She told me to be sure to tell everyone who called how much she appreciated their friendship. I was to thank them for calling, to tell them she was sorry that she had no energy to say hello. I was to remind them to enjoy each day.

With the anger and guilt dissolved, there was now only sadness and my tears, as the house grew quiet and Mom slept most of each day.

Thank goodness she was just down the hall, making it easy for me to look in on her, twenty, thirty, forty--even fifty times a day. I knew she was comfortable and not in pain. I knew she was cared for and loved. I would walk quietly down the hall and stand in her bedroom door, now watching her sleep, just as forty-six years earlier she had stood in mine and watched me asleep in my crib. I loved her so much.

During the last few weeks Mischief spent most of her time sleeping on Mom's bed, close to her legs, giving her extra love and comfort. Our journey became more difficult, but despite it all, I loved Mom being in my home.

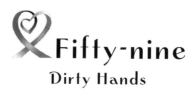

Fifty-nine

Dirty Hands

It was inevitable. With Mom no longer able to get out of bed, the day had finally arrived when she needed diapers. "Dirty hands" is how my girlfriend refers to this stage of caregiving. Knowing all I do today, I would choose to care for Mom again. The good far outweighed the bad, but "dirty hands" is an appropriate phrase.

Caregiving is more than just giving medicine, meals, and baths. It isn't for the faint of heart. Yet with the help from hospice and friends, with prayers and patience, I kept my promise.

Diapers. Neither Mom nor I discussed the impact of this role reversal that screamed "time has passed." I was dreading that moment, but as with so many other moments, when it arrived it was not so bad. I had to make a joke about it, because I literally didn't know what to do. I don't have children and must be one of the few people who had never put a diaper on a baby.

Talking helped lighten the moment. Mom directed me, telling me which side was up, how the sticky tabs on the sides hooked over. Together we figured it out. I was actually embarrassed when the hospice nurse came to care for Mom because my first attempt was far from perfect. But over time, I got better.

I thought Mom might not like me putting on her diaper, but I think I was wrong.

I believe she found it comforting to have her daughter cradle, protect, and take care of her as she did for me when I was a baby. Love and caring is what an infant needs when it starts its life journey. If you're lucky, love and caring is also there as your life journey ends.

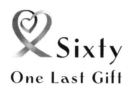

Sixty

One Last Gift

O n March 10, 1999, Mom slipped into a coma. In her case, that meant that she was sleeping or deeply resting around the clock. The experts claim that hearing is the last sense to depart, and they encourage you to speak to a comatose person as you would if you knew they could hear you.

Julie was amazing in her care for Mom. If I was downstairs while Julie was upstairs caring for Mom, I could hear Julie on the Adult Monitor. She would give Mom advance notice of her every action, each word spoken with a soft, loving voice. Julie's voice was soothing to me, and I am certain it was also comforting to Mom.

"Hello Anne, it's Julie," she would say. "How are you doing today? I'm going to rub some lotion on your feet, okay? Now I'm going to turn you on your left side—if it's okay with you."

By the time Mom entered the coma stage, I was forced to acknowledge she would soon pass. She was sleeping around the clock. Her breathing was deep and raspy. It was extremely difficult, but I started to accept it was time for her journey to end. I asked Gay, the hospice chaplain, to come once more and joined her as she gave Mom a blessing and prayed with me.

Due to the guidance and support we received from hospice, we had been blessed with extra time to say our good-byes, to laugh, love, and share. But even in her coma, during what was, for me, a horribly sad time, I received one more miracle. I believe this last gift was possible because Mom was in my home, comfortable, and properly cared for with the guidance of hospice and the others on our team.

I had gone to work that day, since it was one of the days Julie came to the house. At the office, I received a phone call from Dave and Adele, Mom and Dad's dear friends, calling to tell me that they had set a wedding date. The two were going to be married on May 23 in Kauai. They would fly their immediate family to Kauai for the wedding and asked me to join them. I can't tell you how honored I was to be standing in for Mom and Dad. I was very happy for the two of them, and I was selfishly happy because I knew that in a few months I would have the opportunity to enjoy, once again, the beauty of Hawaii.

I was so excited to get home to tell Mom the good news. I knew that she would be happy for Dave and Adele. I ran up the stairs and sat on the chair next to her bed, then made myself comfortable. Mischief was already on the bed lying next to Mom. Pumpkin jumped onto my lap.

"Hi Mom, I'm back home from work. It was another busy day at the office, but I have really great news. Adele called to tell me that she and Dave are getting married on May 23 in Kauai, and they've invited me to join them!"

In the quiet of that moment, I witnessed a miracle: I saw Mom's right fist raise a few inches off the bed. I know, without a doubt, that she heard my every word. In her mind she raised her right arm and pumped her fist to show her excitement and pleasure for Dave and Adele.

I was surprised and amazed, and I was filled with gratitude that Mom heard and understood me. One more memory, one more gift.

Sixty-one

Mom was now wearing long-lasting morphine patches on her back to help keep her comfortable, and she also needed other medication every four hours. She hadn't eaten for a few weeks and hadn't taken in fluid for days. I was mentally and physically exhausted and had hired Sallie, also a nurse, to help care for Mom. Both Julie and Sallie had keys to the house, coming and going as needed. Much of my caregiving was now passed to the experts who were trained to care for a comatose body in the final stage of dying.

It was the day before spring, another day of rain. The weather outside was gloomy and gray, mirroring the mood inside.

Earlier in the week, without thinking, I had picked up an extra blanket lying at the foot of Mom's bed and thrown it around my shoulders. Like Mom, I continued to lose weight, my nervous energy consuming far more calories than the small amounts of food I had eaten that week. I seemed to get colder with each passing day and found the weight of the blanket comforting. I was now in the habit of wearing the blanket throughout the house; it was nice having something to hold onto. I looked silly, but my physical appearance was the last thing on my mind.That afternoon and evening, I sat downstairs in the leather recliner Dad used to enjoy, alone with my thoughts. Missing him, reflecting on our life's recent seismic shift, I stretched out, my feet resting on the footstool, chair reclined for napping, wrapped in my blanket.

Time passed slowly; hours seemed like days, with the silence interrupted by Mom's loud, irregular, raspy breathing. Praying that her spirit would be released from her decaying body, part of me hoped I would not hear another breath, yet I was relieved when I did.

Pumpkin joined me for a few hours, taking a nap on my lap. Mischief was sleeping next to Mom, protecting her. Twice that day, I heard first Julie and then later Sallie come in, say hello, care for Mom, then say good-bye.

Looking out toward the bay, I could see people walking by, holding their umbrellas. In the past few months, I had become familiar with six of them. In the mornings there were the gray-haired lady with her limping collie and the middle-aged man, always smoking a pipe, leading his aging dog. In the afternoons I usually observed the heavy-set lady with the basset hound and the older gentleman with the curved back, who moved with a deliberate but slow pace (as if still walking his long deceased dog). The young couple who walked the small dog with the white curly hair must have been part of the work force since they walked after dark, except for an occasional day appearance on a weekend.

Wondering about their lives, I found some comfort in observing their routines. Did they have a loved one at home? Did they care for a person with an illness? Did they receive the same joy from their pets as I did mine? Did they appreciate their ability to leave home and enjoy a daily walk?

Some days, they would pass in rain gear; other days, they were bundled in winter car coats, their necks wrapped with scarves. They had no idea that inside the house they passed daily a spirit was awaiting its release, a heart was breaking, a loved one departing.

During the "Last Months," three of my friends had become grandparents, two had started new careers, and one had fallen in love. When taking the time to talk with my friends, I encouraged them to enjoy each day to the fullest. Soon it would be time for me to do the same.

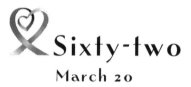

Sixty-two
March 20

At two in the morning I woke up and walked slowly and quietly down the hall to Mom's room. I stood in her bedroom doorway, listening to her erratic raspy breathing, taking one last look at the person I loved more than anyone in the world. Although I still didn't want to let her go, I knew that Mom's time on this earth was nearing an end, and I finally agreed it was time. There was no need to turn on a light; the routine of caregiving needed no further illumination. I gave Mom her medication, ran my fingers through her hair, leaned over and kissed her forehead.

With a broken heart, I whispered, "Thanks for being my Mom. I love you."

I turned, and for the first time, I closed her bedroom door.

I slowly walked back to my bedroom and lay on my bed, tears streaming down my face. Instinctively I knew she was leaving me. I dozed off, waking again about half past six. I was not surprised there were no sounds of life coming through the Adult Monitor. I didn't need to open the bedroom door that morning; I knew she was gone. I don't know how I knew, but I knew.

I walked downstairs and brewed a full pot of strong coffee. Although it was not yet seven that

Saturday morning--Julie's time to be with her family--I called to tell her Mom was gone.

"Oh my," Julie gasped. "Are you okay? Do you want me to come over?"

"I'm okay," I whispered. "I'll call hospice; they'll take care of everything. I just wanted you to know how much Mom and I appreciate all you've done for us. Thank you from the bottom of my heart."

I poured my first cup of coffee, then sat down to call hospice. They said they would send out a nurse in the next hour. Peggy was off that day, so it would be a nurse I had not yet met. I said that was okay and hung up the phone, still numb in my sorrow.

I sat alone at my small kitchen table, sipping coffee, petting the kittens, waiting for the minutes to pass until I could start making phone calls. It was too early to start sharing the sad news.

Hearing the doorbell ring, I opened the door expecting to find the hospice nurse. Much to my surprise, there stood Julie, a stethoscope hanging around her neck.

"I had to come see her one more time," she said, shutting the door behind her as she entered the hall. She reached out with open arms to give me a hug. I was so grateful for everything Julie had done for Mom and for me, especially for rushing to be with me this lonely morning. The moment we touched, I burst into tears that soon turned into heartfelt sobs. Touching Julie reminded me how precious a touch can be; knowing my beloved Mother and I would never again share a caressing touch was a reality too painful to acknowledge.

Only after my tears receded did Julie walk upstairs to see Mom. She stayed with her until the hospice nurse arrived. Together they made phone calls and did the things they are required to do when a patient dies.

Before Julie left, we savored one last hug. As Julie headed out the door, I asked for her hand. In her palm I placed Mom's small emerald ring, purchased by Dad in Mexico during one of their cruises. I knew that Mom would be happy that I had given Julie her ring. I could not have helped Mom in the comforting and loving way that Julie helped her. At first she protested, but by looking in my eyes she could tell that I wanted her to have that ring. That was the last time I saw Julie, but I will always remember the gift of care she gave my mother.

Later that morning, after eight cups of coffee, numerous telephone calls, and hugs from my loving neighbor Anitah, I was joined by the hospice nurse, who came downstairs and sat with me at the kitchen table. She told me that someone from the funeral home would be arriving soon. She let me choose whether or not I wanted to watch them carry out Mom's body. I was grateful for the choice, and let her know that I had already said my good-byes. I walked into my bedroom to take a shower.

After more tears and a hot, twenty-minute shower--a feeble attempt to rinse away my grief--I slipped on jeans, a T-shirt, a sweatshirt, and thick socks. Looking into the mirror at my weary face, I brushed my hair, brushed my teeth, and decided there was no need for make-up that day.

Leaving my bedroom I paused, uncertain if I was ready to enter her room. Looking down the hall, I could see the kittens were already there; after all, that had been our routine for the past four months. I walked slowly down the hall, stopped before entering, then stood in the doorway of Mom's bedroom. The early morning light drew my eyes to the outside tree's first blossom, then eerily bounced off the only items remaining in the now empty room: two nightstands, the bookcase, and one dining chair, with Mom's favorite picture album resting on its cushion. Hospice had dealt with the funeral home and arranged for the removal of the hospital bed, tray, wheelchair, portable commode, walker, raised toilet seat, shower chair, extra diapers, and medications.

My promise kept, I turned and walked away. My life without Mom had begun.

♡ Sixty-three

That afternoon, my voice hoarse from hours on the phone calling her friends and my body shaky from too many cups of coffee, my neighbor and I made a fire in the fireplace. The kittens welcomed the heat, as did I. For a few minutes, Anitah and I sat in silence on the floor in front of the fire, mesmerized by its flickering lights and crackling log.

With tears welling again, I stood and walked into the kitchen; I pushed aside the magnets holding the DNR form on the refrigerator. With my right thumb and forefinger, I grasped the form's top right corner, carried it to the living room, and gingerly placed it on the floor beside me.

Anitah and I bowed our heads and held hands. Our first prayer was of gratitude for the hospice team and the support they provided to Mom and me. Our second prayer of thanks was to Julie, Warren, my colleagues, and friends for taking care of us. Next, we prayed for Mom and for Dad.

Then we offered that damned DNR form to the fireplace god. We watched the form quickly disappear as it was engulfed by flames. I had waited a long time for this moment.

Imagine that, my first smile of the day.

Epilogue

In April 1999, I drove to Southern California, where in the city of Costa Mesa at the lovely home of Mom's cousin, seventy friends and family members joined together to celebrate Mom's life.

The next day, I drove to the desert to see Grandma, wondering whether I should tell her that her daughter had died. I arrived at her assisted living home just before lunch, finding her in her room, dressed and sitting on her couch, looking through her memory box of pictures. After a loving, long overdue hug, I asked to join her for lunch. Together we walked to the dining room, where we were given a table for two by a window overlooking the portico. I shared segments of the past few months, and with tears and trepidation, I told her that Mom had died. Given Grandma's dementia, her only words surprised me.

"Oh honey," she said, "if it's hard on me, I can't imagine how difficult it must be for you." Then Grandma changed the subject and never again mentioned Mom.

I visited with her the following day before driving home, and in the following months, flew to the desert to visit her once a month.

I worked twelve-hour days, six days a week and attended hospice bereavement groups, which were especially helpful in getting through my first birthday, Mother's Day, and Father's Day without my parents. Slowly, I once again started to appreciate the gift of life.

Walking into my office early one weekday morning in August, I noticed that the red message light on my phone was blinking. I was stunned to hear that someone from Eisenhower Hospital in Palm Desert had called the prior evening to tell me that my Grandmother had fallen and broken her hip. She needed surgery right away, and my permission was required. I immediately called the hospital, and after speaking with a doctor, approved the surgery.

It was déjà vu to be calling Alaska Airlines, booking a seat on the afternoon flight from San Francisco to Palm Desert, packing my laptop and urgent work papers, driving home to pack a few clothes, finding someone to watch the cats, and then leaving for the airport. By five that afternoon, I was holding Grandma's hand in her hospital room on the third floor, a place I knew all too well from visiting Dad there the prior November.

At age ninety-seven, Grandma survived the surgery. Unfortunately, her assisted living facility wasn't structured to provide her with the detailed care she now needed, so I had to move her to a nursing home. The hospital social worker provided me with a list of nursing facilities in the area, and I visited several before selecting the one I liked best, one that fit her slim budget.

A few days after Grandma's surgery, I followed the ambulance that took her to the new facility where she would share one small room containing two twin beds, two televisions, and one bathroom. The nursing home provided Grandma's daily physical therapy, but due to her dementia, she couldn't remember to put her weight on one side when she stood. Therefore, she was soon confined to a wheelchair and no longer able to walk. I hated having to leave her, but after a week I needed to go back to the office.

Fortunately, I had several friends in the desert who arranged their schedules so that someone visited Grandma daily, and the following month I flew back as often as I could. Grandma always recognized me and enjoyed being wheeled outside or getting her hair done.

During my visit in late September, while I was helping Grandma eat, she surprised me by closing her mouth, looking me directly in the eye, and shouting "No!"

The next day at breakfast, she repeated her actions, adamant that she no longer wanted to eat. Grandma's health care directive clearly stated that she didn't want a feeding tube. After discussing the matter with the facility, I told Grandma that I would honor her choice. If she wanted to eat, she could; if she didn't want to, that was her decision.

The only good news was that this time I knew where to seek help, or so I thought. After a few days of Grandma not eating and sleeping around the clock, I called hospice. Someone came to evaluate her, but I was told that her heart was strong, she didn't have a life-threatening illness, and thus she did not qualify for hospice.

Four days later, she still had not eaten and had accepted very little water. I again called hospice, explained her current condition, and asked if they would please come re-evaluate her. They agreed, and when they came and saw that her condition had changed, she was accepted into hospice that day. This time, having Grandma's power of attorney, I provided them with her information and signed the necessary paperwork. Even though she was in a nursing facility where she received twenty-four-hour care, hospice sent a nurse to see her, to ensure she was comfortable and not suffering.

A few days later, as the afternoon sun set, I sat next to Grandma's bed, holding her hand as I had held Dad's and then Mom's, and thanked her for being a wonderful, supportive, and fun-loving Grandma. I told her how much I loved her, but that I would be okay if she wanted to leave and be with Mom. She didn't say anything; she just lay in bed with her eyes closed. But I knew she was listening to me, so after leaning over to kiss her good-bye, I whispered, "See you tomorrow Grandma."

The next morning, before the sun rose, the phone rang. I knew the call was about Grandma, and I was right; she joined her daughter early in the morning on October 11, 1999, at the age of ninety-seven.

By the time I dressed and drove to the nursing home, hospice had arrived. As before, they comforted me, explained that they would be sending Grandma's body to the funeral home and handling other details that accompany any death. This time, I knew how many death certificates to order, what to ask, and what to expect.

It had been a most difficult journey, and it would take me more than a few years to move through my sorrow. Collectively, Mom, Dad, and Grandma had been the center of my universe.

Later that year, good friends set me up on a blind date. They introduced me to a wonderful man. Upon learning that I had lost my parents, and after listening to my story, he said, "I'm so sorry. You'll move through your pain and grief, but you will never get over the loss." He spoke from experience. He had lost his father to Lou Gehrig's disease, and then much later also lost his mother, who died of a heart attack, after suffering for seventeen years when a stroke paralyzed her left side.

On our first date, Dave opened the car door for me, pulled out the chair when I sat down at the restaurant, and made me laugh throughout the evening. He was easy to be with and I found myself thinking about his words for several days. I was thrilled when he asked me on a second date. We fell in love, and he became my best friend. We were married on the tenth anniversary of our first date, and we will both be forever grateful to our friends who arranged that blind date.

Life, filled with joy and sorrow, is constantly changing. My husband likes to say, "All days are good; some are just better than others."

Rae Ann McKeating

Acknowledgments

First and foremost, thank you to my husband Dave. From the day we met you have understood my heart's desire to share my story and help others learn the benefits of hospice. I am extremely grateful for your patience, love, and support the past ten years while I worked on this project. You never complained about the thousands of hours I spent writing and rewriting at the dinner table. When I was ready to quit, you let me take a break, then at the right time you encouraged me to keep trying. You are an incredible partner and I'm lucky to be your wife.

My heartfelt thanks to Jacque Burton for designing the double-heart ribbon book cover and chapter image (*www.jacqueburton.com*); to Lynn Campbell for your professional expertise; to Tiffany Nichols for your photographic skills; to the members of the Southern California group, Write-On, who helped me more than you will ever know, and to Leslie Ryan for your support and for sharing the knowledge you gained after publishing your first book.

Special thanks to my friends and family; you each energized me along the way. Your words and support have been invaluable.

A personal thank you to Joe Perrone Jr., a published author who put down his pen, donned his editor's hat, and turned my words into a book.

Finally, I cannot imagine taking my family on its end-of-life journey without hospice. To both hospices, the Visiting Nurse Association of the Inland County in Palm Desert, now known as VNA California, and Hospice of Marin, now known as Hospice by the Bay, I owe so much. I have shared my story so others will know about hospice, should they find themselves on a similar journey. I will forever be grateful for the invaluable care and support hospice provided us.

Thank you for taking the time to read my story. If you have any thoughts, questions, or would like to share your hospice/caregiving experience, please visit me on my website at *www.endoflifeissues.com.*

Made in the USA
San Bernardino, CA
19 January 2015